COVID-19

THE GENETICALLY ENGINEERED PANDEMIC

Peter Tremblay

Dr. Orion Zee, Ed. and Foreword

Agora Books

Agora Books™
Ottawa, Canada

Agora Books$_{TM}$
P.O. Box 24191
300 Eagleson Road
Kanata, Ontario K2M 2C3 CANADA

Agora Books is a self-publishing agency for authors that was launched by The Agora Cosmopolitan which is a registered not-for-profit corporation.

ISBN: 978-1-927538-74-6

Printed in Canada

Book cover art
General Art Work, by Raymond Samuels [Front cover]

CONTENTS

CONTENTS

FOREWORD

I STAND BEFORE YOU AS a physician and a scientist who has both a passion for facilitating the health & wellness of people, as well as the truth. Unfortunately the official narrative on the COVID-19 pandemic is a lie. Similarly, the official story that vaccines are being developed around the world that will save us all is also untrue.

We are being fed blatantly false and misleading information regarding testing, case numbers, mortality, and the use and effectiveness of masks, lockdowns, and potential therapies.

No vaccine has ever been successfully developed to immunize against any natural coronavirus. Indeed, it is apparent that COVID-19 was genetically engineered to mutate in ways which make any reliable vaccine impossible. The likelihood that COVID-19 could have originated completely from nature is for all intents and purposes, absolutely zero.

The architects of the pandemic have created and perpetuated totally false hopes in a vaccination program as a salvation for humankind. The real purpose of vaccination programs around the world appear to be to draft humans as guinea pigs for miscellaneous medical experiments which have nothing to do with immunization.

This book pulls together evidence to support the premise that we are being misled by well financed groups which operate across national boundaries.

The physicians and scientists who have sought to turn a blind eye to the medically obvious nature of COVID-19 as having been genetically engineered, knowingly or unknowingly participate in the betrayal of humans to an unspeakable evil.

When I became a doctor, I did not seek to sell my soul for a mess of pottage.

The protection of democracy relies on the free flow of information which will enable citizens to make rational choices.

Democracy has not been served by efforts both within and beyond the medical-scientific establishment to repress the true source of the prevailing pandemic.

It is my personal and professional view that humanity's best hope to combat the genetically engineered pandemic should not focus on the cynical direction of vaccination but instead start with the natural enhancement of human immune systems, the use of well-known time-tested therapies, and the focused protection of the elderly and the vulnerable.

I can say to you in good conscience that evil people run the world and they are who is behind this pandemic. I ask you to keep an open mind. Scrutinize not only information but the very source. Seek the truth. Protect each other, and be eternally vigilant.

—Orion Zee, M.D., Ph.D.

PREFACE

THE REAL CONSPIRACY THEORY OF the pandemic is the idea that it was the result of a lack of acceptable hygiene standards in a Chinese market. As revealed by investigative researchers and whistleblowers like Dr. Li-Meng Yan, the reality of the pandemic is that COVID-19 was concocted in a laboratory to deal with what its engineers viewed as a "problem."

While many people think that conservation and protection are the best way to deal with a growing environmental crisis, this view does not appear to be shared by many others, including elites. For many elites, the central focus of the global environmental crisis, along with the worsening scarcity of natural resources, is a soaring world population.

For such elites who don't want to change the capitalist economic status quo, the solution is, therefore, not the spreading of social justice and the legislation of strong environmental regulations, but instead to reduce the world's population through the spreading of diseases that will "cull the human herd" of society's "weak and inferior." Therefore, the genetic engineering of COVID-19 represents a pragmatic approach to dealing with a future that elites fear and want to better control.

These elites believe humans ought to be managed with the same ruthless approach that would be applied to managing and taming any animal population that has gone "out of control" relative to the environment's ability to safely sustain that animal population. Whereas in agriculture, this approach has been referred to as animal husbandry, in society, this approach, which elites have sought to embrace, is called eugenics.

This ideology can be readily seen in how elites allowed the pandemic to spread globally through disinformation. Similarly, it is visible in how elites have allowed the pandemic to ravage extended care facilities and various oppressed minority communities that are collectively viewed by elites to be from the "weak" or "inferior" populations that COVID-19 was meant to target in the first place. That is why the sympathy expressed by elites has not been matched with the kind of action that could easily work to contain COVID-19 within the communities that have been hit the hardest by the pandemic.

The repression of the truth about COVID-19 that Dr. Yan and other scholars have sought to reveal is a testament to the ability of the rich and powerful who support the eugenics goals of COVID-19 to use that power to subvert the free flow of information that would expose their oppressive agenda against humanity.

COVID-19 represents nothing short of a crime against humanity, and those who have concocted it present a substantive and immediate threat to the future of humanity as a sovereign species with free will on Earth. COVID-19 seems to be a step in unveiling a plan for a significantly reduced world population that is put under the control of a totalitarian global order modelled from Chinese authoritarianism that will be controlled by artificial intelligence (AI) enabled through the delivery of a biometric vaccine program. This vaccination program is not speculation but is already being implemented in parts of the so-called "third world," where "banana republic" governments have been co-opted by elites to use human guinea pigs to test out a biometric roll-out planned for the rest of the world.

As Dr. Yan revealed in her interview with Brian Rose on LondonReal, the creation of a vaccination to treat the constantly mutating biogenetic weapon COVID-19 is not plausible. The vaccination, therefore, does not offer a cure, as the masses have been fooled to believe, but simply a ruse to implement another phase by the elites to control and reduce the human population through "infertility" and human DNA re-sequencing. Vaccination trials have apparently enabled this to go forward and expedite humanity toward a "New World Order" AI grid.

In the article entitled "Twilight of the Psychopaths," Kevin Barrett wrote:

Civilized people, we are told, live peacefully and cooperatively with their fellows, sharing the necessary labour in order to obtain the leisure to develop arts and sciences. And while that would be a good idea, it is not a good description of what has been going on in the so-called advanced cultures during the past 8,000 years. Civilization, as we know it, is largely the creation of psychopaths.

All civilizations, our own included, have been based on slavery and "warfare." Incidentally, the latter term is a euphemism for mass murder.

The prevailing recipe for civilization is simple:

1) Use lies and brainwashing to create an army of controlled, systematic mass murderers;

2) Use that army to enslave large numbers of people (i.e. seize control of their labour power and its fruits);

3) Use that slave labour power to improve the brainwashing process (by using the economic surplus to employ scribes, priests, and PR men).

Then go back to step one and repeat the process.

Psychopaths have played a disproportionate role in the development of civilization, because they are hard-wired to lie, kill, injure, and generally inflict great suffering on other humans without feeling any remorse.

The inventor of civilization—the first tribal chieftain who successfully brainwashed an army of controlled mass murderers—was almost certainly a genetic psychopath. Since that momentous discovery, psychopaths have enjoyed a significant advantage over non-psychopaths in the struggle for power in civilizational hierarchies—especially military hierarchies.

With that said, it is apparent that the COVID-19 pandemic represents the most recent chapter in human history of an event carefully planned by psychopaths.

Humanity's best hope to recover from the prevailing pandemic does not lie in vaccines, which are part of a psychopathic orchestration, but by we, as humans, collectively elevating our consciousness toward a service-to-others focus that will enable us to interrupt a demonic alien matrix which has sought to push us towards an ego-driven service-to-self focus.

The insatiable pursuit of power that has become an inextricable part of human society is the very basis for the genetic engineering of COVID-19. As humans, we have legitimated hierarchies of power that have conditioned elites to see the genetic engineering of COVID-19 as a logical response to dealing with "overpopulation," which, in their view, will lead to an anarchy they cannot control, and such an anarchy is a threat to their power.

The idea that COVID-19 was genetically engineered is, therefore, not some sort of farfetched "conspiracy" but a perfectly understandable reaction by psychopaths, which is not only consistent with human history but the evidence this book now presents.

In writing *COVID-19: The Genetically Engineered Coronavirus Pandemic*, I hope to contribute to efforts to rejuvenate approaches to dealing with the pandemic and help prevent our planet from descending into global totalitarian control by a clique of insiders and a regressive alien-controlled artificial intelligence matrix. Not only is the future of our planet at stake, but the very survival of humanity as a sentient species with free will that is guided by a soul that embraces empathy, peace, and love. It is apparent that the architects of the COVID-19 pandemic seek to replace the human species we are now with a robotic version of humans under their complete control and direction.

WHO MADE THE COVID-19 VIRUS?

WHAT IS THE TRUE SOURCE of the Wuhan coronavirus? Thanks to intentional disinformation that's spread through the mainstream media, many members of the public have resigned themselves to the thought that they may never know the source of the novel coronavirus, or why the virus was bioengineered by the world's dominant powers.

In December 2019, several cases of pneumonia with unknown cause developed in Wuhan, Hubei, China, and these cases all resembled viral pneumonia. However, upon further investigation by scientists who took lower respiratory tract samples of the early patients, the virus was found to be one that hadn't been seen before; subsequently, it was named the 2019 novel coronavirus, also often referred to as COVID-19, 2019-nCoV, and SARS-CoV-2.[1] As time went on, cases of the virus began to spread from China to Thailand, Japan, South Korea, the United States and the rest of the world—and, as to be expected, people started to panic.

During this time, Donald Trump, the president of the United States of America, suggested he had seen evidence that the 2019 coronavirus originated in a Chinese laboratory. President Trump had been answering questions from journalists at the White House, and a reporter had asked: "Have you seen anything at this point that gives you a high degree of confidence that the Wuhan Institute of Virology was the origin of this virus?"

"Yes, I have. Yes, I have," President Trump had replied without hesitation. "And I think the World Health Organization [WHO] should be ashamed of themselves because they're like the public relations agency for China."[2]

Chinese supreme leader Jinping Xi quickly denied any accusations that his country may have bioengineered a virus, either knowingly or unwittingly, that escaped from the lab, but in a contradictory move, he called an emergency meeting, after which China issued directives to all the bioengineering labs in the country to follow stricter protocols.[3]

Steven W. Mosher, president of the Population Research Institute, noted that the directive issued by the Chinese government to its labs is suggestive of guilt,[4] while other scientists wondered if it were a mere coincidence that the only Chinese lab equipped to handle advanced viruses such as the novel coronavirus is located in Wuhan.

Others pointed to the fact that a top biological warfare expert in the People's Liberation Army, Major General Wei Chen, was redeployed to Wuhan at the end of January 2020 to help with the effort to contain the outbreak. Chen was well-known for her work in researching coronaviruses since the 2003 SARS outbreak, and she was sent to the bioengineering lab in Wuhan to help contain the virus—the same lab from which the virus was said to have escaped.[4]

While these events are somewhat strange, is this enough evidence to conclude that China unleashed a killer virus on its own population? Or is the United States of America just pointing a finger at China because a finger was first pointed at them?

What about the possibility that the dominant Western powers (America and its allies) engineered a biological attack on China in a combined attempt to contain her growing influence? At first, this may seem farfetched, but there exist possible reasons why the United States would potentially launch a deadly engineered biological attack on China.

For one, it is important to consider the fact that ever since the "Trump trade war," the Chinese people and even their livestock have faced several hazardous and lethal germs, viral diseases, and illnesses in usually lethal strains that threatened to cripple the Chinese people, their food, and their livestock.[5]

It was widely speculated that the Trump administration had, prior to the COVID-19 pandemic, been relentlessly deliberating on the topic of growing Chinese global competitiveness and how this growth threatens American national security and economic dominance. It's therefore not difficult to see how one may suspect that the Trump administration may have created and unleashed the virus in one of its efforts to crash China's thriving economy and her military.

Interestingly, a remarkable event took place in October 2019, when the Johns Hopkins Center for Health Security, in conjunction with the World Economic Forum and the Bill and Melinda Gates Foundation, held a meeting of American military leaders, NEOCON political figures, and various other world leaders of business, government, and public health to simulate a situation in which a coronavirus pandemic was wreaking havoc on the planet. Many people found it strange that the Chinese were not invited to this meeting, even as most major viral disease outbreaks in recent years have occurred in Africa and China.

The day after this meeting, 300 U.S. military personnel went to Wuhan for the Military World Games on October 19.[5]

Fourteen days later, on November 2, 2019, the first coronavirus case was seen in Wuhan. Remarkably, fourteen days is also the total incubation period for the coronavirus. This is not to say for a fact that the U.S. military personnel brought the virus into China, even though many have this suspicion. There is also the issue of China's top virology lab being located in Wuhan and how the virus may have been fabricated in that lab. While there are obvious and valid reasons for these suspicions, governments and the mainstream media have made it almost impossible for people to ask these questions. Anyone who speaks out on the topic of the bioengineered COVID-19 virus is quickly labelled a conspiracy theorist, while research on the topic of bioengineering of the COVID-19 virus is never acknowledged by the mainstream media. Why is this?

WHY WOULD ANYONE
MANUFACTURE A LETHAL VIRUS?

A CCORDING TO DAVID E. MARTIN, Ph.D., a national intelligence analyst and owner of IQ100 Index (NYSE), in 2003, just after the SARS outbreak in Asia, the U.S. Centers for Disease Control and Prevention (CDC) saw the potential of a gold strike with the coronavirus. They had discovered, during the 2003 SARS pandemic, that the virus could be easily manipulated and therefore could be extremely profitable. So, in 2003, they sought to patent the virus and they made sure that they held the proprietary rights to the virus, its detection, and all the measurements of it. The CDC, led by people like Dr. Anthony Fauci, controlled 100 percent of the cash flow that built the empire around the industrial complex of the coronavirus.[6] On April 25, 2003, the CDC filed a patent for the coronavirus that's transmitted to humans.

Interestingly, under Title 35 U.S. Code Section 101,[7] nature is prohibited from being patented; therefore, it is either the COVID-19 virus was manufactured, thereby making the patent legal, or the virus is natural, thereby making the patent illegal. In either outcome, the CDC would be in the wrong.[8]

Therefore, it is not surprising that, in 2007, the CDC filed a petition with the patents office to keep their patents private. This means that the CDC can, at the moment, control who can or can't make independent enquiries on the virus. Not everyone is allowed to look at the virus, measure it, or develop a test kit for detecting it. By getting a patent that constrained anyone else from using the virus, they had the means and motive to turn the virus from a pathogen to a profit venture. Today, developing and owning a coronavirus vaccine has become like the gold rush.[6]

From 2013–2014, the National Institutes of Health (NIH) suspended gain-of-function (GOF) research on coronavirus, arguing that there was no reason to make a virus more dangerous than it already is. The federal funding for research that usually goes to great institutions such as Harvard and the University of North Carolina was stopped. The NIH had a moral, social, and even legal reason to stop this kind of research. Yet, the letters sent to researchers clearly stated that the government was cutting off funding for this kind of research but researchers were free to continue conducting this kind of research voluntarily.[6]

In 2014, when the heat for failing to completely stop this kind of research started getting to the NIH, they offshored the research out of the country, to the Wuhan Institute of Virology (WIV).[9] Dr. Anthony Fauci, the current director of the National Institute of Allergy and Infectious Diseases, came along and made it possible for the research money on gain-of-function research to be diverted to Wuhan. The continuation of this kind of research led to the formation of COVID-19.

Prior to the outbreak of the COVID-19 virus, the United States channelled all grant money for GOF research to China, but they did not give these grants directly; rather, they ran the money through a series of organizations, which then subcontracted these projects to the WIV.

Secretary of State Mike Pompeo has already been on record confirming and defending this funding, claiming that the reason for the funding was "to protect American people from labs that aren't up to standard."[10]

Did the United States divert all their GOF research to China so that, when caught, the USA could blame China and China could blame the USA and no one would ever know who was indeed responsible for creating the killer coronavirus? Sound familiar?[2] The cruel part is that both countries are almost telling the truth, but not everyone is buying into what the governments are claiming.

Meryl Nass, M.D., a physician, writer, and researcher, was the first person in the world to ever look into a pandemic and discover that it had been bioengineered. Nass wrote a paper twenty-eight years ago titled "Anthrax Epizootic in Zimbabwe 1978–1980: Due to Deliberate Spread?" From the onset of the COVID-19 pandemic, Nass stated she never believed that the virus could have occurred naturally from bats. She was convinced that the virus is a lab-designed pathogen.

Nass spoke about a paper dated March 17, 2020 published in *Nature Medicine*, that claimed the virus was certainly a natural occurrence. The paper, titled "The Proximal Origin of SARS-COV-2"[11] offered several arguments that made no scientific sense, yet many important scientists started parroting the claims of this paper. Nass says she wondered why these people were risking their reputation making these illogical claims about the 2019 coronavirus and concluded that someone must have made those five scientists publish that article and someone must have convinced other scientists to agree with them.

In an interview, Nobel laureate, medical researcher, and virologist Professor Luc Montagnier was quoted as saying about the new coronavirus: "It was a meticulous job, done professionally." He insists that the job must have been done by an expert in the field and does not at all appear natural, claiming there is an uncanny amount of precision found in the virus sequence, too precise to be the handiwork of nature.[6]

All the evidence regarding the bioengineering of the virus has been brought to light since the onset of the epidemic, but the mainstream media and most Western governments prefer to push their own narratives for their own profit. When fact-checkers confront the powers that be with evidence of the virus's bioengineering, they're labelled conspiracy theorists and made to feel like they're transgressing. True information about the virus has been heavily censored, while giant search engine Google tries to ensure that searches on the topic of bioengineering of the COVID-19 virus only bring up one side of the story—the side that favours the CDC. Google creates the illusion that numerous sources have concluded the same thing about the virus, with no dissenting voice. But in reality, Google has hidden all research on the topic that opposes popular belief.

The illusion of unanimity on the topic emboldens the public to share the CDC's chosen narrative as the truth, when in reality, the public is being used to push propaganda.

Scientists Prove That the Virus Was Bioengineered

The authors of a British–Norwegian vaccine study published by the *Quarterly Review of Biophysics* identified "inserted sections placed on the Sars-CoV-2 Spike surface." According to the three scientists who published this study, the virus uses these artificial insertions to attach onto cells. They confirmed that the COVID-19 virus was "significantly different from any SARS we have studied."[12] According to these researchers, 21.6 percent of the composition of this coronavirus' spike protein is made up of nonhuman-like (NHL) epitopes.

The study further revealed that these insertions, which the scientists called synthetically controlled "chimera", were created in the Wuhan virology lab and did not occur naturally, as many had been led to believe. The report indicated that the virus was fully adapted in the lab before it was launched to the rest of the world.

This study was released in Cambridge University's *QRB Discovery* by University of London professor Angus Dalgleish and Norwegian virologist Birger Sorensen.

Sorensen told Norwegian reporters that it is "rather unusual for infections that cross species barriers," and that the novel coronavirus has structural properties that are very different from SARS and "which have never, ever been spotted in nature."

The scientist stated that he strongly believed the virus was a product of "gain-of-function studies" that had been going on in China. It is worth noting that many countries conduct "gain-of-function studies," and that the United States and China have been performing such research for years.

SCIENTISTS HAVE MANUFACTURED VIRUSES IN THE LAB FOR YEARS

WHEN IT COMES TO VIRUSES, gain-of-function research aims or expects to increase transmissibility and/or virulence. This is the medical process used in adulterating viruses.[13] Gain-of-function research studies produce the virus in the lab so it can be duplicated more easily to carry out multiple clinical research studies.

In GOF research, a new virus is intentionally made, either through in-vitro mutation or by cutting and joining two or more viruses. The aim of such reconstruction is to make viruses more deadly by adding novel functions such as amplified infectivity or pathogenicity. Experiments are then carried out on these new viruses, either in cell cultures or in whole animals. This class of experiments was banned in the United States from 2014 to 2017.

Another major high-risk experiment carried out in laboratories to make new viruses is known as passaging. Passaging requires putting a live virus in an animal or cell culture to which it is not adapted, and then, while the virus is still alive, transporting it to another animal or cell of the same type. The aim of passaging is to let viruses evolve rapidly and become adapted to new animals or cells.

One of the most well-known investigations on passaging was carried out in the lab of Dutch researcher Ron Fouchier, who took an avian influenza virus (H5N1) that was non-contagious in mammals and serially passaged it in ferrets. His aim had been to create a potential pandemic pathogen (PPP). After they had done 10 passages, the scientists realised that the virus had indeed progressed—not only was it infecting ferrets but it was transmitting to others in neighbouring cages. In this way, scientists created an airborne ferret virus.[14]

Some researchers have been known to combine gain-of-function studies with passaging experiments by using recombinant viruses in passaging experiments.[15]

In 2015, scientists investigated a virus called SHC014, which is found in horseshoe bats in China. The researchers created a chimeric virus, made up of a surface protein of SHC014 and the backbone of a SARS virus that had been adapted to grow in mice and to mimic human disease. This study was published in *Nature Medicine* in November 2015.[16] This particular study triggered renewed debate over whether engineering lab variants of viruses with possible pandemic potential is worth the risks.

In the paper, the scientists who conducted the study agreed that these kinds of studies were sometimes deemed unnecessarily risky. "Scientific review panels may deem similar studies building chimeric viruses based on circulating strains too risky to pursue," they write, adding that discussion is needed as to "whether these types of chimeric virus studies warrant further investigation versus the inherent risks involved."[16]

"The only impact of this work is the creation, in a lab, of a new, non-natural risk," said Richard Ebright, a molecular biologist and biodefense expert at Rutgers University in Piscataway, New Jersey, and a longstanding critic of gain-of-function studies.

Aside from these experiments, viruses can be genetically engineered and have often been engineered to be used as vectors to deliver functional genes (or gene inactivation) in gene therapy to treat genetically inherited diseases. For instance, there are oncolytic viruses that are programmed to kill cancer cells and stop tumours from spreading.

Other examples of genetically engineered viruses include the development of live attenuated vaccines for preventing viral infections. There are also ongoing clinical attempts to boost B-cells to produce antibodies against dangerous viruses that currently do not have any vaccines. The foregoing is proof that viruses can indeed be made in the laboratory, but what happens when virus bioengineering goes wrong?

No Virus Resembling COVID-19 Has Been Found in Nature

RESEARCHERS FROM SEVERAL COUNTRIES HAVE confirmed that there is certainly something unnatural about the novel coronavirus.

The mainstream media has stated from the start that the virus came from nature. But they need to answer one question: where is the evidence that the virus indeed came from an animal, as speculated? Indeed, there are no indications that animals are the intermediaries for this virus, nor are there are plausible explanations that explain the natural zoonotic transfer of the COVID-19 virus to humans. There is, however, an abundance of research available that show exactly how scientists produced this virus in the laboratory.

A 2020 investigation published in the *Journal of Antiviral Research* sequenced the genome of the virus and promptly released its genomic information. The six-man study concluded that, "Despite a high similarity with the genome sequence of SARS-CoV and SARS-like CoVs, we identified a peculiar furin-like cleavage site in the Spike protein of the 2019-nCoV, lacking in the other SARS-like CoVs."[17]

One researcher explains the process used by scientists in identifying virus sequences: "Viruses are essentially comprised of a nucleic acid core surrounded by a protein coat. The protein coat contains specific glycoproteins that enable them to bind to receptors in the body causing them to fuse to the cell membrane and release their nucleic acid sequence to infect the cell. The virulent nucleic acid sequence hijacks the cellular machinery to self-replicate, lyse the cell, spread, and infect other cells. Using reverse genetics, the sequence of a viral genome can be identified, including that of its different strains and variants. This enables scientists to identify sequences of the virus that enable it to bind to a receptor, as well as those regions that cause it to be so virulent."[18]

After studying reports on the sequences of the virus, the ex-head of the British Secret Intelligence Service (MI6) Sir Richard Dearlove told journalists that he believed the novel coronavirus had been bioengineered. "I do think that this started as an accident," he said. "It raises the issue, if China ever were to admit responsibility, does it pay reparations?"[19]

More Details on Why the COVID-19 Virus Could Not Have Come from Nature

WHILE MANY SCIENTISTS HAVE MAINTAINED that all evidence points towards the fact that the virus was certainly bioengineered in a lab, it is interesting how much effort certain governments and institutions have made towards silencing anyone who claims to have proof that SARS-CoV-2 was genetically engineered.

From the onset of the pandemic, early reports claimed that most COVID-19 cases seem to have occurred in and around Wuhan's Huanan Seafood Market; however, recent research finds that many of the earliest cases did not originate from the animal market.[1]

Interestingly, the Chinese Foreign Ministry official Lijian Zhao does not believe that the virus came from the market; he insisted that the U.S. Army brought the virus to China. This enraged U.S President Trump and other top officials, who denied these allegations.

The United States Director of the National Institute of Allergy and Infectious Diseases and a key adviser to Mr. Trump on the pandemic, Dr. Anthony Fauci, denied that the virus could have come from either the United States or from a Wuhan lab.

His reason? "If you look at the evolution of the virus in bats and what's out there now, [the scientific evidence] is very, very strongly leaning toward this could not have been artificially or deliberately manipulated," he said.[20] "Everything about the stepwise evolution over time strongly indicates that [this virus] evolved in nature and then jumped species."

However, if you look at the evidence available, then Dr. Fauci couldn't be more wrong about the virus evolving from nature because one troubling factor remains, which scientists have never quite been able to explain, and that is the fact that Wuhan city, the epicentre of the COVID-19 pandemic, also happens to be the global epicentre of bat coronavirus research.[21] Based on this one intriguing fact, many felt quite strongly that there is a chance that the virus may have a laboratory origin. Many scientists feel that one of the labs in Wuhan known for their research on coronaviruses may have either intentionally released a bioengineered virus or accidentally let one escape.[22]

Even though many factors about the origin of the virus remain disputed among scientists, a majority agree that the nearest known relatives to the COVID-19 virus are found in bats. This is the reason many researchers have erroneously concluded that the COVID-19 virus must have also come from bats.[23]

However, these 'close relative' bat coronaviruses in question do not have the capacity to infect humans.[24] Therefore, from the onset of the pandemic, many wondered how a bat RNA virus could evolve into a human pathogen that is not only contagious but also deadly.

Reporters and scientists have tirelessly mulled over scenarios by which the natural zoonotic transfer of the virus may have occurred. Some researchers tried to explain this puzzle by blaming a likely intermediate species. Snakes, civets, and pangolins were mentioned as likely temporary hosts. The two preceding coronavirus near-pandemics of SARS (2002–2003) and MERS (2012) were both suspected to have come from bats and then transitioned to humans via intermediate animals (civets and dromedaries, respectively), so many assumed that the COVID-19 virus may have evolved in the same way.[11]

Since bat coronaviruses never possessed an ACE2 cellular receptor (the molecule which allows cellular entry of the virus), and this receptor was found to be a major part of the COVID-19 virus, these scientists claim that this bridging animal that served as a temporary host to the virus would probably have been intermediate in protein sequence (or at least structure) between the protein sequence of bats and humans.[25] However, all these are assumptions, with no scientific proof; meanwhile, there is an abundance of proof in favour of bioengineered viruses.

A History of Lab Releases

THE 1918 INFLUENZA PANDEMIC, ONE of the most severe pandemics in recent history, was caused by an H1N1 virus with genes of avian origin. The virus is estimated to have infected about one-third of the world's population. At least 50 million worldwide died from the virus. One interesting feature about this virus was that it killed young and healthy people. Death rates were high among those less than 5 years old, those 20–40 years old, and those 65 years and older.

The CDC will confirm that even though the 1918 H1N1 virus has been synthesized and evaluated, the properties that made the virus so overwhelming are not well understood.[26]

H1N1 affected countries worldwide, with a large number of people suffering globally, until everyone began to build immunity to the now so-called extinct virus. Although the CDC would say that there is no universal consensus regarding where the virus originated,[26] other researchers insist that, in 1977, a laboratory in Russia (or possibly China) accidentally released the H1N1 influenza virus while trying to make a vaccine for the flu.[27]

It is worth noting that HIN1 broke out again in 2009–2010 and was renamed "swine flu," causing an estimated 3,000 to

200,000 deaths.[27, 28] For obvious reasons, the virology community has been hesitant about discussing these topics.[29, 30]

Aside from H1N1, other laboratory pathogens have led to human and animal deaths. For instance, smallpox once broke out from a lab in Britain, and equine encephalitis escaped from a lab in South America.[31] These incidents have now become so common that the world ought to have more information about them than is currently available.[32]

Many scientists have cautioned that experiments with potential pandemic pathogens, like the smallpox, Ebola, and influenza viruses, are fundamentally dangerous and should be subject to strict limits and oversight.[33, 34]

The Indian defence establishment believes the 1994 Surat Plague is a case of bioterrorism. Numerous media outlets at the time reported the involvement of the American Centers for Disease Control and Prevention (CDC). It was suspected that the germ, with an extra protein ring, was developed by a CDC lab in Almaty, Kazakhstan.[35]

Researchers report that, since the end of the SARS outbreak in 2003, there have been six documented SARS disease outbreaks originating from research laboratories, including four in China. These outbreaks caused 13 individual infections and one death. [32] As discussed earlier, to forestall such outbreaks, in 2014, the United States banned gain-of-function studies with potential pandemic pathogens (PPPs); this ban was in the form of a funding moratorium.

Instances abound in history where viruses have escaped high-security labs in various forms. Most laboratory incidents causing exposure to pathogens in high-security labs in the United States were caused by human error and sometimes equipment failure.[36]

A 2004 SARS outbreak in China was traced back to the country's National Institute of Virology (NIV) where there had been an inadequate inactivation of a viral sample that had been distributed to parts of the building that were not secure.[37] Likewise, a U.S. Defense Department laboratory once claimed to have mistakenly sent live *Bacillus anthracis*, the bacterium that causes anthrax, to nearly 200 laboratories worldwide in a 12-year period. The laboratory said they had assumed that the samples had been inactivated. Again, in 2007, a foot-and-mouth disease outbreak in Britain originated from the malfunctioning waste disposal system of a BSL-4 laboratory leaking into a stream from which neighbouring cows drank.[32]

To cut a long story short, pathogens have been leaking from laboratories for many years now, many times undetected or accidentally uncovered and most times underreported. So it is important to examine the chances that the bioengineered COVID-19 virus may have escaped from the lab.

Based on the reasons above—and to ensure the safety of humanity by preventing future man-made pandemics, or at least be prepared for it—it is crucial that world governments ignore toxic politics, establish the true source of past pandemics, and at least make genuine efforts to confirm whether the laboratory-escape hypothesis has credible evidence to support it.

Did Dr. Zhengli Shi Make the 2019 Coronavirus?

Wuhan, China, is the hometown of the Wuhan Institute of Virology (WIV), China's first and only Biosafety Level 4 facility. This is the highest pathogen security level facility obtainable. This highest-level lab, which had only just been added to the WIV in 2018, has been collecting large numbers of coronaviruses from bat samples ever since the initial SARS outbreak of 2002–2003, including additional collection in 2016.[38; 39]

These projects were led by top coronavirus researcher Zhengli Shi, and some of them involved experiments in which live bat coronaviruses were introduced into human cells.[38]

Besides being the home of the biggest virology institute in the country, Wuhan is home to a lab known as the Wuhan Centers for Disease Prevention and Control (WCDPC). This lab is only about 250 metres from the Huanan Seafood Market, and is a BSL-2 lab that has, in the past, been used to house bat coronaviruses.

So the question on many people's lips became: Did scientists from one of these labs, under instructions from a higher authority, unleash this virus on the world for an ulterior purpose? Did researchers from one of these Wuhan labs get infected with a SARS-CoV-2-like bat coronavirus on one of their several virus-collecting trips, also called virus surveillance trips? Or, maybe a virus that was being studied or manipulated in one of the labs escaped?

The safety of the WIV, which was built in 2015 and commissioned in 2018, has been examined several times in the past years. Josh Rogin of *The Washington Post* once reported that U.S. Embassy officials visited the WIV in 2018 and afterwards warned their superiors in Washington of a "serious shortage of appropriately trained technicians and investigators needed to safely operate this high-containment laboratory." *VOA News* also reported that "a security review conducted by a Chinese national team found the lab did not meet national standards in five categories."[31]

Chinese officials have also raised some concerns about biosafety in the past after visiting the lab. In 2019, Zhiming Yuan, a biosecurity specialist, wrote on the issues faced by such facilities in China and noted that China intended to build more labs in the near future. He wrote: "Several high-level BSLs have insufficient operational funds for routine yet vital processes," and "Currently, most laboratories lack specialized biosafety managers and engineers." He recommended that "We should promptly revise the existing regulations, guidelines, norms, and standards of biosafety and biosecurity."[31]

One of the most prominent voices with solid scientific evidence on the topic of the bioengineered COVID-19 virus is an anonymous scientist. Many scientists who spoke out about the SARS-CoV-2 virus in the early days chose to do so anonymously based on the fact that there are powerful interests and emotions

surrounding the virus. It is also known that Chinese scientists
were forbidden to speak publicly about the virus while the disease
ravaged their cities. Therefore, it is difficult to ignore important research from scientists who may have chosen to remain
anonymous to ensure their own safety.

The anonymous scientist who runs an anonymous blog called
Nerd Has Power, utilized scientific evidence and logical thinking
to evaluate, and legitimize, the possibility that the 2019-nCoV,
SARS-2-CoV virus is of non-natural origin.[40]

The scientist, referred to hereafter as "Nerd," strongly contends that the bat coronavirus (RaTG13) that scientists claim is
the so-called natural source of SARS-CoV-2 is nothing but a
mere fabrication. Nerd asserts that the powers that be fabricated
a natural origin for the virus so that the people responsible for
creating the COVID-19 virus would not be punished.

The author accused Zhengli Shi, director of the Wuhan Institute of Virology in China, of being responsible for bioengineering the virus. According to Nerd, "The WIV is only a few
kilometres from the Wuhan seafood and wildlife market that
was initially blamed for the outbreak. Shi has been dubbed by
the media 'the bat woman' for her role in collecting bat viruses
from the wild for her 'gain-of-function' research." As a renowned
coronavirus expert in China, Zhengli Shi has always been suspected of creating this virus, which was then let out of the lab,
either accidentally or on purpose.

Nerd clarifies that the reason many people are suspicious of
the origin of the COVID-19 virus is also due to how the sequence
(genome) of this virus compares with other related coronaviruses.

Comparing the Sequence of the COVID-19 Virus to Other Coronaviruses

G ENOMES ARE COMPARED EITHER BY comparing their gene sequences or the protein sequences they encode. Viral genomes only encode for a limited number of proteins. According to Nerd, a virus is known to typically produce a single polyprotein by translating its entire genome and then cuts this long polyprotein at specific places to produce a set of particular proteins for specific use. Therefore, he compared different viruses based only on their protein sequences.

This comparison revealed that the 2019 coronavirus is about 86% identical to the SARS coronavirus of 2003. This could only mean that the 2019 coronavirus does not have the same origin as the 2003 SARS virus; most scientists would agree to this.

On the other hand, there are two other viruses that have a weird resemblance to the 2019 coronavirus. These are bat coronaviruses, namely ZC45 and ZXC21. On comparing them with these two bat coronaviruses, Nerd concludes that, "Overall, the sequence of either of the two bat coronaviruses is 95% identical to the Wuhan coronavirus. In fact, for most part of the genome, such level of identity is maintained or even surpassed. The E protein, in particular, is 100% identical. The nucleocapsid is 94% identical. The membrane protein is 98.6% identical. The S2 portion (2nd half) of the spike protein is 95% identical. However, when it comes to the S1 portion (1st half) of the spike protein, the sequence identity suddenly drops to 69%."

Not only is the above pattern of sequence conservation between the viruses in comparison extremely rare, it is also exceptionally strange. Nerd explains that natural evolution typically takes place when mutations occur unsystematically across the entire genome. You would then expect the rate of mutation to be more or less the same for all parts of the genome.

Nerd admits, however, that such strange patterns of sequence identity could be caused by other forms of evolution. Recombination is one evolutionary event that could lead to drastic changes in only one part of the genome. However, Nerd explains in his article that recombination would have been practically impossible in this case.

To begin proving the bioengineering of the virus, Nerd starts off by analysing the S1 portion of the spike proteins—the protrusions outside the virus—shown below.

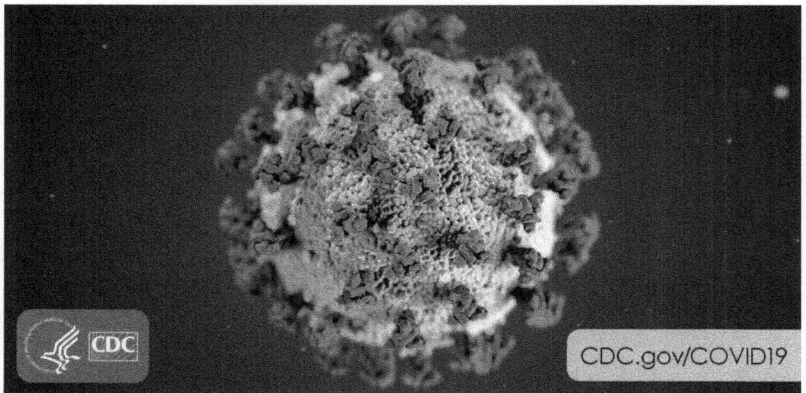

Figure 1. A model-generated image of the coronavirus particle with spike proteins (red) decorating its surface. Image adapted from the CDC website.

Spike proteins serve as the keys with which coronaviruses unlock human cells to gain entry into the body.

It is worth noting that while the COVID-19 virus looks almost identical to its bat relatives (ZC45 and ZXC21) everywhere else, it differs in appearance when it comes to its S1 spike proteins. Interestingly, the S1 spike protein is the protein responsible for viruses binding the host receptor. In Nerd's words, "S1 can be considered as the portion of the 'key' that literally enters the 'lock.' It has to fit precisely to the delicate shape of the 'lock' (host receptor) so that the 'door opening' action can be accomplished. Whether or not a particular 'lock' can be opened by a specific 'key' is decided exclusively by this S1 part of [the] spike." In other words, S1 of a coronavirus dictates whether a virus would infect humans or not.

The S1 spikes in the bat coronaviruses ZC45 and ZXC21 are incompatible with, and thus cannot bind to, human receptors, which is the reason these coronaviruses have not been responsible for any pandemics. Surprisingly, the COVID-19 virus failed to inherit the incompetent S1 spikes in the harmless viruses that it otherwise resembles in every other way. Rather, the COVID-19 virus somehow possesses the same short-piece S1 spike from the SARS virus. Thanks to this strange replacement in S1 in which all key residues were preserved and many non-essential residues were altered, COVID-19 has the ability to infect humans, unlike its brother bat viruses.

A recent publication confirms that the spike protein of the SARS virus and the coronavirus look pretty much the same;[41] however, in spite of this evidence, many scientists blame this similarity on natural evolution and recombination. These scientists ignore all evidence and insist that there is no basis for this claim, as studies have proven that the virus is naturally evolved.

One article in particular states: "Sequencing the genome of the SARS-CoV-2 virus have revealed that it is a beta-corona-virus of lineage b and contains a furin-like cleavage site which is absent in lineage b coronaviruses including the closely related SARS-CoV. This is what led to some media outlets suggesting that the presence of this additional element in the virus suggests that it was tampered with or modified in a way to make it more dangerous."

This researcher claims that the strange cleavage site found on the virus is simply a part of the virus's initial host. "Furin-like enzymes are present in most mammals and birds, and the presence of the furin-like cleavage site indicates that the virus was originally hosted in another animal, but once it evolved to infect humans, it still contained this cleavage site which allows it to spread more efficiently in humans. This is simply an obser-vation of virus evolution (natural recombination), and scientists cannot just simply attach a functional cleavage site to a virus in this manner."[18]

Nerd, however, contends that these alterations are too precise to be the handiwork of nature. Even though the spike proteins of different coronaviruses often differ, greater discrepancy in S1 spike proteins are only often observed when two viruses have been long detached during evolution and have adjusted, through random mutation, to their hosts for a very long period of time. In his words, in cases where this happens, "The overall sequence identity would be low as well. In the present case, however, the sequence identity between either of the bat coronavirus and the Wuhan coronavirus is over 95%, suggesting these two viral lineages must have diverged from each other fairly recently. Therefore, a sequence identity of 69% for the S1 portion of spike protein is simply insane."

More important to this topic is another bat coronavirus called the RaTG13. Many scientific publications that support the notion that the virus comes from nature rely on the single piece of evidence that the sequence of the COVID-19 virus is over 90 percent identical to the RaTG13 virus.[42]

Several scientists who have had the chance to examine an image of RaTG13 report that it looks almost like the 2019 coronavirus throughout the whole sequence of the viral genome. Since these scientists assume that RaTG13 is a natural virus, they immediately conclude that COVID-19 must also be natural, seeing as they have already identified its common ancestor. The only problem with this assumption is that the RaTG13 virus is not a real virus.[40]

Interestingly, Shi, China's "Batwoman", also happens to be the person who first reported the sequence of RaTG13. Shi was nicknamed "Batwoman" for her work capturing wild bats in caves to detect and isolate coronaviruses within them. The aim of her research was to find those coronaviruses that were likely to cross over from bats to humans because she intended to help the world avoid another pandemic like SARS in future.

However, rather than carry out her self-proclaimed mission, it seems Zhengli Shi created a virus that almost destroyed nations.

As the COVID-19 outbreak intensified and people began to point fingers at Shi, she immediately published a paper.[39] In the paper, Shi likened the sequence of the Wuhan coronavirus to that of other coronaviruses, and therefore, she defined an evolutionary path for COVID-19. It was in this paper that Shi reported the RaTG13 virus to the world for the very first time. In other words, the RaTG13 virus, which had been unheard of for years, all of a sudden and out of nowhere, in the middle of the

COVID-19 pandemic, appeared and almost shaped a consensus in the field that the COVID-19 virus originated from nature.

In Shi's paper, she stated that RaTG13 was discovered in Yunnan province, China, in 2013. It has been alleged by credible sources that Shi has admitted to not possessing a sample of this RaTG13 virus. According to Shi, her lab had only collected bat feces in 2013 and found the sequence information of the virus during their research . . . which means that there is no real proof that the RaTG13 virus exists. All the information that is known about this virus is nothing but a string of letters. Because of this, Nerd argues that this RaTG13 virus could easily have been fabricated.

Nerd, writing in his blog, states, "It takes a person less than a day to TYPE such a sequence (less than 30,000 letters) in a word file. And it would be a thousand times easier if you already have a template that is about 96% identical to the one you are trying to create." He goes on to describe how easy it could be for a scientist to release false data to the world: "Once the typing is finished, one can upload the sequence onto the public database. Contrary to general conception, such database does not really have a way to validate the authenticity or correctness of the uploaded sequence. It relies completely upon the scientists themselves – upon their honesty and consciences. Once uploaded and released, such sequence data becomes public and can be used legitimately in scientific analysis and publications."[40]

Nerd has just one question for anyone who does not believe RaTG13 is fake. Since Shi claims she discovered the virus in 2013, why did she wait seven whole years to share the information with the world, especially since the sequence of the RaTG13 virus is highly alarming and clearly shows a potential to infect humans?

Shi came into the limelight in 2013 with her discovery of two bat coronaviruses, Rs3367 and 9SHC014, which are similar to SARS.[24] It is worth noting that this was the work that proved, for the first time, that SARS originated from bats. Since 2013, her team has published a series of important information about these coronaviruses [43, 38] and nothing about the RaTG13 virus. If RaTG13 was indeed a real virus, why did Shi go through lengths to keep it hidden from the public?

Furthermore, the WIV team insists it did not create the virus, but since the 2003 SARS outbreak, they had never stopped working on potential pandemic pathogens (PPPs).

In reality, the WIV had been involved in an intensive search for SARS-like pathogens since 2004, and is known for its collection of bat coronaviruses.[44] It has gone on several collecting trips since its original one in 2004.[45]

Through gain-of-function studies, Shi's team was performing dangerous experiments using these collected viruses. In 2013, the Shi lab reported isolating an infectious clone of a bat coronavirus, which the team named WIV-1.[46] The team obtained this virus by introducing a bat coronavirus into monkey cells, passaging it, and then testing its infectivity in human (HeLa) cell lines engineered to express the human ACE2 receptor.[46] The WIV team was conducting these experiments even until recent years.

Shi also was once the co-author of a paper that performed GOF research on bat coronaviruses.[47]

"In 2017, again with the intent of identifying bat viruses with ACE2 binding capabilities, the Shi lab at WIV reported successfully infecting human (HeLa) cell lines engineered to express the human ACE2 receptor with four different bat coronaviruses. Two of these were lab-made recombinant (chimeric) bat viruses.

Both the wild and the recombinant viruses were briefly passaged in monkey cells."[38]

These projects served one major purpose: to find out whether an advanced pathogen could break out from the wild by creating them in the lab.

An Independent Science News stated "The Shi lab collected numerous bat samples with an emphasis on collecting SARS-like coronavirus strains, 2) they cultured live viruses and conducted passaging experiments on them, 3) members of Zheng-Li Shi's laboratory participated in GOF experiments carried out in North Carolina on bat coronaviruses, 4) the Shi laboratory produced recombinant bat coronaviruses and placed these in human cells and monkey cells. All these experiments were conducted in cells containing human or monkey ACE2 receptors."[31]

The aim of these WIV experiments was to engineer pathogens with pandemic potential to test the likelihood of similar coronaviruses breaking out in the future to cause pandemics.

Consider the fact that almost every scientific publication since the outbreak of the COVID-19 pandemic seems intrigued by the fact that the virus has a unique feature never before seen in similar viruses—the spike protein that binds with exceptionally high affinity to the human ACE2 receptor "at least ten times more tightly" than the older SARS viruses.[48, 49, 50]

This high affinity is remarkably absent in other animals such as snakes, pangolins, and civets, yet exceptionally present for humans, which further proves the point that the COVID-19 virus is a pathogen highly adapted to humans.[51] Considering the fact that the WIV lab has a research and collection history on coronaviruses, it is not at all far-fetched to want to explore the possibility that the COVID-19 virus may have been trained up on the human ACE2 receptor by passaging it in cells expressing that receptor.

The WIV lab has also been known in the past to amplify spike proteins of collected coronaviruses,[52] which would make them available for GOF experimentation.

Many researchers have sought to throw more light on the fabrication of this virus, and to make the public aware of the level of science going on right under our noses.

One researcher insists that every virology lab in the world that has ever conducted a genomic analysis of the coronavirus knows that the coronavirus was engineered by human scientists. [19] This researcher insists that there are some sequences that just cannot occur by chance in nature and says that the tools that were used for genetic insertion in the coronavirus are still present as remnants in the genetic code and anyone who examines the virus closely could find this.

According to the researcher, the WHO and the CDC are covering up the bioengineering of this virus in order to protect China's biological weapons program because no government wants the public to know the full truth about how frequently government-run labs experience outbreaks.

Dr. Yuhong Dong, who holds an M.D. from Beijing Medical University and a doctorate in infectious diseases from Beijing University, also confirmed that the virus could not have occurred in nature.[53]

In Dong's words, "Based on recently published scientific papers, this new coronavirus has unprecedented virologic features that suggest genetic engineering may have been involved in its creation. The virus presents with severe clinical features, thus it poses a huge threat to humans. It is imperative for scientists, physicians, and people all over the world, including governments and public health authorities, to make every effort to investigate this mysterious and suspicious virus in order to elucidate its origin and to protect the ultimate future of the human race."

The doctor refers to a science paper published in *The Lancet* on January 30 that concludes "recombination is probably not the reason for emergence of this virus." In other words, this did not occur through natural mutations in the wild.[54]

Dong also reminds the world of a study by five Greek scientists published January 27, 2020 that found that the coronavirus has no lineage to other viruses in the "family tree" that's found in the wild.[54]

Not to mention the January 2020 *Lancet* study that found that no bats were sold or found at the Huanan Seafood Market around the time of the outbreak of the COVID-19 virus.[54]

"First, the outbreak was first reported in late December 2019, when most bat species in Wuhan are hibernating. Second, no bats were sold or found at the Huanan seafood market, whereas various non-aquatic animals (including mammals) were available for purchase. Third, the sequence identity between 2019-nCoV and its close relatives bat-SL-CoVZC45 and bat-SL-CoVZXC21 was less than 90%. Hence, bat-SL-CoVZC45 and bat-SL-CoVZXC21 are not direct ancestors of 2019-nCoV."

Experts from institutions all over the world echoed the need for further research on the origin of the virus but they were ignored.[55]

Evidence from the Nikolai Petrovsky-led Study

In April 2020, four scientists from the Australian Science Media Centre were asked to investigate whether the COVID-19 virus indeed came from the lab. The study was led by a virologist from Flinders University named Nikolai Petrovsky. Petrovsky told the Media Centre that "no natural virus matching to COVID-19 has been found in nature despite an intensive search to find its origins."[56]

Nikolai Petrovsky, a professor in the College of Medicine and Public Health at the university, concluded that "While SARS-CoV-2 has some similarities to SARS CoV and other bat viruses, no natural virus matching to COVID-19 has yet been found in animals."

Petrovsky explains how his group of scientists at Flinders University, in collaboration with researchers at La Trobe University, studied the possible evolutionary origins of COVID-19 by modelling interactions between its spike protein and a wide range of ACE2 receptors from animals and humans.

Their research[51] revealed that the strength of binding of the COVID-19 virus to human ACE2 surpasses the predicted strength of binding to ACE2 of the other tested species. Petrovsky concluded that there was something peculiar about the virus that needed further investigation; in his words, "This high binding to human ACE2 suggests the possibility that the COVID-19 spike protein has previously undergone selection on human ACE2 or a closely related ACE2 variant. How this might have happened is currently unknown and warrants further scientific investigation."

Subsequently, Petrovsky told reporters that he suspects human manipulation in Wuhan because of the unmatched ability of the virus' protruding spike to infect human cells.

"This, plus the fact that no corresponding virus has been found to exist in nature, leads to the possibility that COVID-19 is a human-created virus," said Petrovsky. "It is therefore entirely plausible that the virus was created in the biosecurity facility in Wuhan by selection on cells expressing human ACE2, a laboratory that was known to be cultivating exotic bat coronaviruses at the time."

A laboratory-treated coronavirus also could have escaped the facility through an accidental infection of a staff member who then visited the Wuhan wild animal market, Petrovsky said. Other potential sources include inappropriate disposal of medical waste at a Wuhan laboratory or transmission from a cat or other animal that came into contact with infected waste.

According to Petrovsky, the rapid evolution of the coronavirus and its exceptional capacity to infect humans is either "a remarkable coincidence or a sign of human intervention."

"While COVID-19 has close similarities to SARS and other bat viruses, no natural virus matching to COVID-19 has been found in nature despite an intensive search to find its origins," he elaborated. "This raises the very legitimate question of whether the COVID-19 virus might be the result of human intervention."

Even though the Australian study, alongside other studies, couldn't easily find signs of artificial gene inserts that would signal virus engineering, Petrovsky explained that there are ways to engineer viruses without such inserts. For instance, laboratory technicians could take a bat coronavirus that is not infectious to humans and force its evolution by culturing the virus with cells that have the human receptor. That process was used to culture SARS coronaviruses in laboratories. The result would be that "you can force the bat virus to adapt to infect human cells via mutations in its spike protein," Petrovsky said. Laboratory development of viruses can also create other random mutations.

"The result of these experiments is a virus that is highly virulent in humans but is sufficiently different that it no longer resembles the original bat virus," he said.

Since those mutations would be acquired randomly in a laboratory, there would be no signature of bioengineering, Petrovsky explained, "but this is clearly a virus still created by human intervention."

The Petrovsky-led study concludes that the binding energy of the virus' "spike" protein is at its highest for humans and greater than for all other species tested, including bats, which is the most suspected likely original source. (The team analysed a range of animals, such as civets, pangolins, hamsters, mice, dogs, cats, snakes, tigers, cows and horses.)

"This indicates that SARS-CoV-2 is a highly adapted human pathogen," concludes the Australian report. "Overall, the data indicates that SARS-CoV-2 is uniquely adapted to infect humans, raising important questions as to whether it arose in nature by a rare chance event or whether its origins might lie elsewhere."

In his statement, Petrovsky goes on to describe the kind of experiment that, in principle, if done in a lab, would obtain the same result as the hypothesised natural zoonotic transfer and rapid adaptation of a bat coronavirus to a human host.

Other scientists publicly agreed with the findings of this Australian study. For instance, Jonathan J. Couey, a research assistant professor of neurobiology at the University of Pittsburgh, spoke to reporters, stating that, while understanding the origin of the virus is extremely important to finding a cure, debate on the lab origin of the virus has been slowed down by scientists opposed to even considering the possibility of a lab origin.[57]

"Understanding the exact origin of this virus is vital to ensure that all scientific and medical data are interpreted correctly by policymakers and health care professionals alike," he told the media, going on to assert that "Several scientists with obvious conflicts of interest have been permitted to go on the record denying that it would be possible to generate such a virus in a laboratory and stating specifically that the sequence of SARS-CoV-2 would never have been chosen by any 'gene jockey.'"

Conclusively, Couey said, "Both of these denials are not genuine scientific rebuttals, but rather semantic pseudo-denials formulated by some of those most closely tied to the funding of these [gain of function] research lines."

Other researchers have found four insertions in the spike glycoprotein of the virus. It was confirmed that these insertions have not been present in any other past coronaviruses. They also found amino acid residues in all the inserts that closely resembled the key structural proteins of HIV-1 and which they concluded were unlikely to have been accidentally formed in nature.[58]

Despite the fact that many public and private researchers have advised that it may be fatal to dismiss the possibility of an accidental laboratory leak of the COVID-19 virus, and that knowing the origin of the virus could prove critical to finding vaccines and treatments and responding to future outbreaks, U.S. intelligence agencies have only so far continued to maintain that they agree with a "wide scientific consensus" that the virus evolved from nature. They stated this in an April 30, 2020 statement by the Office of the Director of National Intelligence.

The Australian study is only one of the several scientific papers to suggest that a laboratory manipulation played a part in the evolution of the virus.

A group of Indian scientists published a paper in January 2020 that was later withdrawn when the publication faced pressure from China. This withdrawn study had found that the COVID-19 virus contained four insertions to the spike protein that are unique to SARS-CoV-2 and not found in other coronaviruses. The researchers admitted that these insertions looked oddly similar to those found in the HIV-1 virus and the scientists concluded that these features were "unlikely to be fortuitous in nature."[58]

Even though the paper was withdrawn under pressure from China, the scientists involved in the study have refused to repudiate their research and promised to publish their findings eventually.

The Chinese government's secrecy on the issue at the beginning of the outbreak also raised eyebrows. At first, the Chinese government insisted that the virus had first originated in the Huanan Seafood Market in Wuhan, but later changed its official version to say the origin is something for scientists to study. Chinese Foreign Ministry spokeswoman Chunying Hua insisted that the Wuhan Institute of Virology could not have been the source of the outbreak. The head of the Wuhan laboratory has also said she is convinced, after a review, that her lab played no role in the virus' spread.

This same government had also initially opposed international calls for an investigation into how the disease outbreak began but later bowed to pressure, stating that it would support an independent WHO probe of the handling of the disease outbreak at an unspecified date.

The attempt by the Chinese to shroud the COVID-19 virus in mystery prevented scientists from learning about the virus; this inquiry into the nature of the virus was needed the most at the onset of the outbreak.

According to Petrovsky, "The nature of this event and its proximity to a high-risk biosecurity facility at the epicenter of the outbreak demands a full and independent international inquiry to ascertain whether a virus of this kind of COVID-19 was being cultured in the facility and might have been accidentally released."

The study by Petrovsky's team challenges the assertions by other scientists that there is no evidence that the virus is the result of laboratory bioengineering.

Another study concluded that contemporary research has failed to fully account for all possible origins of two unique genomic characteristics found in the COVID-19 virus.[59] The study encouraged scientists to look into the long history of serial passage as a method to manipulate viral genomes. The paper states, "The long-standing practice of serial passage is a form of gain-of-function research that forces zoonosis between species, and requires the same molecular adaptations necessary for a natural zoonotic jump to occur within a laboratory, leaving the same genetic signatures behind as a natural jump but occurring in a much shorter period of time."

The study explores the two distinctive features possessed by the COVID-19 virus. Firstly, it examines the virus' spike protein and its unique sequence in the receptor binding domain (RBD), a region known to be critical for the COVID-19 virus utilization of human angiotensin converting enzyme (ACE2),which is the cell surface receptor used by both SARS-CoV and SARS-CoV-2 for fusion with target cells and subsequent cell entry. Secondly, the study explores the presence of a polybasic furin cleavage site within the coronavirus' novel spike protein that is not found in SARS-CoV or other lineage B coronaviruses. The study describes this furin cleavage site as being made up of "multiple basic amino acids, is an important virulence feature observed to have been acquired by fusion proteins of avian influenza viruses and New-castle Disease Virus either grown under experimental conditions or isolated from commercial animal farms—settings that mimic the conditions of serial laboratory passage."

The research categorically states that while there is no naturally occurring influenza virus with a furin cleavage site, these furin cleavage sites are found within several branches of the coronavirus family tree, but never before has it been found among lineage B coronaviruses (of which the COVID-19 virus is one). The study emphasizes that this topic has been thoroughly investigated in the literature because furin cleavage sites "allow the influenza viruses that carry it to establish a systemic multi organ infection using different cell types including nerve cells, is correlated with high pathogenicity, and also plays a key role in overcoming the species barrier. More generally; despite the fact that not all serially passed viruses have demonstrated an increase in pathogenicity, the fact remains that every highly pathogenic avian influenza virus, defined by having a furin cleavage site, has either been found on commercial poultry farms that create the pseudo-natural conditions necessary for serial passage, or created in laboratories with gain-of-function serial passage experiments."

The only other coronaviruses known to have these furin cleavage sites are only 60% identical to the novel coronavirus at most. For the reasons above, the origin of the COVID-19 virus remain questionable. Add this to the fact that the behaviour of the virus continues to puzzle scientists, and researchers have concluded that "the virus acts like no microbe humanity has ever seen."[60]

Interestingly, influenza viruses with artificial furin cleavage sites are known to cause lymphopenia in infected mice, and to cause neurological conditions in the brains of ferrets; both of these conditions are also observed in hospitalized patients infected by COVID-19.

Scientists have considered the possibility that the novel coronavirus gained its furin cleavage site through recombination in an intermediate host species; however, studies have explained why the COVID-19 virus could not possibly be a product of recombination.

According to Nerd in the post we discussed earlier, "What happens in a recombination event is that one segment of a gene can be "replaced" by a similar segment from another gene. In evolution, recombination events happen much less frequently than random mutations. When recombination happens, however, it often brings abrupt changes to certain areas of the genome."[40]

He writes, "If naturally-occurring recombination event(s) lead to the creation of the Wuhan coronavirus, how would it transpire? First, it would have to take place when an ancestor bat coronavirus, something very similar to ZC45 or ZXC21, co-existed with another coronavirus in the same cell of the same animal. Under extremely rare circumstances, recombination may occur, where a random piece in the ancestor's genome is replaced by a similar but different piece from the other coronavirus. Importantly, to go from such ancestor to the Wuhan coronavirus, one combination event is not enough. What has to happen is that recombination has to take place twice during the evolution of the Wuhan coronavirus. In one occasion, the ancestor bat coronavirus would have to acquire, through recombination with a SARS-like coronavirus, the precise short segment of S1 that is responsible for human ACE2 interaction (region highlighted in orange in both Figure 2 and Figure 3). In another occasion, the 'improved' bat coronavirus would further swap in a furin-cleavage site through recombination with yet another coronavirus that carries a furin-cleavage site between its S1 and S2 of spike."[40]

The most interesting thing about these discoveries is how hard the mainstream media has tried to ignore these studies and their implications. So far, only independent media outlets have dared to report on the topic of bioengineering of the coronavirus, and most of these independent platforms have now been systematically censored from Twitter and other social media platforms and search engines for spreading "misinformation."

The reality is exactly as health activist and owner of NaturalNews.com, Mike Adams, wrote: "Any suggestion that the coronavirus was engineered as a bioweapon had to be immediately eliminated." He continued, "The prevailing panic by the establishment sought to blame this outbreak on Mother Nature – i.e. bats, snakes, seafood, etc. – rather than the human beings who are playing around with deadly biological weapons that are designed to extinguish human life."[61]

In April 2020, Peter Daszak, president of the EcoHealth Alliance, was quoted to have told reporters during an interview that the lab escape thesis was "pure baloney." He said, "There was no viral isolate in the lab. There was no cultured virus that's anything related to SARS coronavirus 2. So it's just not possible."

In another interview, he claimed, "There is zero evidence that this virus came out of a lab in China." He insisted instead that the public blame "hunting and eating wildlife."

The issue when the mainstream media insist on interviewing the likes of Daszak and no one else is that the public never gets to know the truth about the virus. First, Daszak claims that no cultured virus at WIV is related to the COVID-19 virus, yet the closest related known coronaviruses to the virus are at the WIV.

One report considers the possibility that Daszak and Shi could be collaborators and both responsible for the high-risk experiments that went on at WIV for many reasons. First is the fact that Daszak is the named principal investigator on multiple U.S. grants that were granted to WIV. He was also Shi's co-author on numerous papers, including the 2013 *Nature* paper announcing the isolation of coronavirus WIV-1 through passaging.[45] One of his co-authorships is on the collecting paper in which his WIV colleagues placed the four fully functional bat coronaviruses into human cells containing the ACE2 receptor.[46]

For her part, Shi told Scientific American, "I had never expected this kind of thing to happen in Wuhan, in central China." During her research, Shi had found that the southern, subtropical provinces of Guangdong, Guangxi, and Yunnan were at the highest risk of coronaviruses jumping to humans from animals—particularly bats, a known reservoir. Wuhan is not in the list of high-risk centres, which had Shi thinking, "Could they [the virus] have come from our lab?"[62]

From all available evidence, it is clear there is a great chance the virus may have come from the WIV lab, so to ask questions about this is not unreasonable, and to ignore these questions makes it seem like there is more to the story than meets the eye.

THE VACCINATION AGENDA

ANDATORY GENE-ALTERING VACCINES MIGHT JUST be a key to the emerging new world post-COVID-19. On March 18th, Bill Gates took part in an AMA (Ask Me Anything) on Reddit titled "I'm Bill Gates, co-chair of the Bill & Melinda Gates Foundation. AMA about COVID-19," where he answered questions about the pandemic. During this session, Gates referred to a "digital certificate" to keep track of who got vaccinated.[63]

Gates had been asked about the changes to be expected after the pandemic, regarding how businesses will operate to maintain the economy while providing social distancing.

He replied, "The question of which businesses should keep going is tricky. Certainly food supply and the health system. We still need water, electricity and the internet. Supply chains for critical things need to be maintained. Countries are still figuring out what to keep running. Eventually we will have some digital certificates to show who has recovered or been tested recently or when we have a vaccine who has received it."

The mention of digital certificates raised a few eyebrows, with one Reddit user likening Gates's solution to the "Mark of the Beast" mentioned in the Bible.

Taking a stand against mandatory vaccines is now more important than ever, as arguably the world powers have engineered a fake pandemic for the sole purpose of forcing a vaccine on the world.[64]

The introduction of a coronavirus vaccine would be accompanied by a technocratic feature characterized by a currency reset and other features such as new levels of visible surveillance, social credit scores, debt forgiveness, universal guaranteed income, Internet of Things, energy-use quotas, and smart cities.

Interestingly, Dr. Fauci, the director of the National Institute of Allergy and Infectious Diseases, mentioned in the middle of the pandemic that the COVID-19 vaccine could be a DNA vaccine.[65] This means it would be a kind of gene therapy where synthesized genes would be injected into the body to allegedly set up immunity, when in reality, these genes would alter the genetic makeup of the recipient, creating an opportunity to put many different genes into humans in a bid to create "new humans."

These so-called immunity passports or risk-free certificates mentioned by Gates and Dr. Fauci would be issued to people who test positive on the new antibody tests for COVID-19. Since 1984, a negative test has been all that was needed to show a person was not infected for a virus; this begs the question, why the sudden shift?

These immunity certificates are believed to be the beginning of the process of conditioning the population to signify immunity via a certificate. It would function as some sort of passport to the "brave new world"—a license to show that you are immune and permitted to conduct business, travel, or attend school. People who are not immune would be injected with these so-called antibodies.

A March 2015 article published in the *New York Times* references a study on DNA vaccines and the use of synthetic genes to "protect against disease," while changing the genetic makeup of humans.[66] According to the article, "By delivering synthetic genes into the muscles of the [experimental] monkeys, the scientists are essentially re-engineering the animals to resist disease."

The article stated:

"'The sky's the limit,' said Michael Farzan, an immunologist at Scripps and lead author of the new study.

"The first human trial based on this strategy — called immunoprophylaxis by gene transfer, or I.G.T. — is underway, and several new ones are planned." [That was five years ago.]

"I.G.T. is altogether different from traditional vaccination. It is instead a form of gene therapy. Scientists isolate the genes that produce powerful antibodies against certain diseases and then synthesize artificial versions. The genes are placed into viruses and injected into human tissue, usually muscle."

The study noted that the synthetic gene is incorporated into the recipient's DNA, altering the human genetic makeup, which is quite scary. The New York Times explained, "The viruses invade human cells with their DNA payloads, and the synthetic gene is incorporated into the recipient's DNA. If all goes well, the new genes instruct the cells to begin manufacturing powerful antibodies."

The makers of this dangerous technology already expect some sort of resistance from the general public as no one would willingly submit to gene-altering vaccines when their real purpose has not been made clear. The New York Times article quotes accomplished researcher and Nobel prize winner Dr. David Baltimore, stating, "Still, Dr. Baltimore says that he envisions that some people might be leery of a vaccination strategy that means altering their DNA, even if it prevents a potentially fatal disease."[67]

The public must therefore unite and take a stand against any genetic technology that seeks to reinvent the human race.

THE DECEPTION BEHIND COVID-19

THREE INTERVIEWS STAND OUT FROM outspoken scientists who have, against all government efforts to silence them, remained resilient in speaking the truth.

First is the Chinese virologist Dr. Li-Meng Yan, who told Fox News in a July 10, 2020 interview that she believes China knew about the coronavirus well before it claimed it did. She maintained that her supervisors also ignored research she was doing that she believes could have saved lives.[68]

Yan was one of the very first scientists to speak publicly about the deception surrounding the COVID-19 pandemic.

In her interview, she exposed many cover-ups at the highest levels of government and spoke a lot about President Jinping Xi and his Chinese Communist Party's tendency to want to control the coronavirus narrative. She revealed the true information about the virus that was made available to China at the onset of the pandemic, and spoke of how the Chinese government edited the information before disseminating it to the rest of the world.

"The reason I came to the U.S. is because I deliver the message of the truth of COVID," she told Fox News in the interview, adding that if she tries to tell her story in China, she "will be disappeared and killed."

Yan, who worked at the University of Hong Kong, was among the very first scientists in the world to study the COVID-19 virus. She alleges that her supervisor at the University/WHO reference lab, Dr. Leo Poon, had in 2019 asked her to look into the odd cluster of SARS-like cases emanating from mainland China towards the end of the year.

"The China government refused to let overseas experts, including ones in Hong Kong, do research in China," she said. "So I turned to my friends to get more information."

Yan says she was initially chosen to conduct the research on COVID-19 because she had an extensive network of professional contacts in various medical facilities in mainland China, having grown up and completed much of her studies there. Her team felt they were not getting accurate info from the Chinese government and had sent Yan to talk to her contacts.

According to Yan, one of her friends, a scientist at the Chinese Center for Disease Control and Prevention, had personal knowledge of the early COVID-19 cases and had told Yan on December 31, 2020 that there were human-to-human-transmission COVID-19 cases while China and the WHO were still denying that such spread was possible.

When Yan reported these urgent findings to her boss, all she got was a nod, and an instruction to keep working on her research.

Yan was shocked a few days later when the WHO put out a statement: "According to Chinese authorities, the virus in question can cause severe illness in some patients and does not transmit readily between people... There is limited information to determine the overall risk of this reported cluster."

Soon Yan began to notice that colleagues across China who had been otherwise willing to discuss the peculiarities of the novel virus had a sudden change of attitude. Doctors and researchers from Wuhan—the epicentre of the virus—were restricted from granting interviews on the subject.

According to Yan, the doctors said, ominously, "We can't talk about it, but we need to wear masks"

The few sources who still mustered up enough courage to talk to Yan told her that the numbers of human-to-human transmission had begun to grow exponentially.

"There are many, many patients who don't get treatment on time and diagnosis on time," Yan said. "Hospital doctors are scared, but they cannot talk. CDC staff are scared."

Again she reported these findings to her supervisor, who, this time, asked her to be more secretive with her findings. In her words, he asked her "to keep silent, and be careful."

"As he warned me before, 'Don't touch the red line,'" Yan said, referring to the government. "We will get in trouble and we'll be disappeared."

Yan also mentions Professor Malik Peiris, the co-director of a WHO-affiliated lab, whom she said knew about how deadly the virus really was but chose to remain silent. On the WHO website, Peiris appears as "adviser" on the WHO International Health Regulations Emergency Committee for Pneumonia due to the Novel Coronavirus 2019-nCoV.

At this point, Yan got frustrated, even though she expected this kind of behaviour from her government.

"I already know that would happen because I know the corruption among this kind of international organization like the WHO to China government, and to China Communist Party," she said. "So basically... I accept it but I don't want this misleading information to spread to the world."

As was expected, the WHO and the Chinese government have also denied that Yan, Poon, or Peiris ever worked directly for the WHO, and the University of Hong Kong, where Yan had been employed, quickly terminated her employment.

The University of Hong Kong took down her webpage and apparently revoked her access to her online portals and emails, even though she says she was on an approved annual leave. In a statement to reporters, a school spokesperson said Yan is not currently an employee.

"Dr Li-Meng Yan is no longer a staff member of the University," the statement read. "Out of respect for our current and former employees, we don't disclose personal information about her. Your understanding is appreciated."

Similar evasiveness surrounds Peiris. "Professor Malik Peiris is an infectious disease expert who has been on WHO missions and expert groups–as are many people eminent in their fields," WHO spokeswoman Margaret Ann Harris said in an email. "That does not make him a WHO staff member, nor does he represent WHO."

Yan says that, in spite of any pushback, she has been encouraged by a sense of right and wrong and says she had to speak up despite the personal and professional consequences.

"I know how they treat whistleblowers," she said. "I know how they treat whistleblowers."

However, Yan wasn't discouraged; she was determined to speak the truth, and when a U.S.-based Hong Kong blogger tipped her off that her life and the lives of her close family members were in danger, she decided to relocate to the United States and warn the world about the virus.

Yan landed at Los Angeles International Airport after her 13-hour journey and was stopped by customs officials, who interrogated her for hours.

"I had to tell them the truth," she said. "I'm doing the right thing. So I tell them that 'don't let me go back to China. I'm the one who came to tell the truth here of COVID-19... And please protect me. If not, the China government will kill me.'"

The FBI was allegedly called in to investigate. Yan claims they interviewed her for hours, took her cell phone as evidence, and allowed her to continue to her destination.

The FBI told Fox News it could neither confirm nor deny Yan's claims; however, Fox News was shown an evidence receipt that appeared to confirm an interaction.

As Yan was trying to find her footing in America, she says her friends and family back home were being threatened by the Chinese government.

Yan claims the government visited her hometown of Qingdao and that agents turned her tiny apartment upside down and interrogated her parents. When Yan finally got in touch with her parents, they begged her to come home, told her she didn't know what she was talking about, and pleaded with her to give up the fight.

The Chinese Embassy in the United States told Fox News they don't know who Yan is and maintained that China has handled the pandemic heroically.

"We have never heard of this person," the emailed statement read. "The Chinese government has responded swiftly and effectively to COVID-19 since its outbreak. All its efforts have been clearly documented in the white paper "Fighting COVID-19: China in Action" with full transparency. Facts tell all."

The WHO has also continued to deny any wrongdoing during the earliest days of the virus. The medical arm of the United Nations has been taken to task recently by scientists challenging its official view of how the virus spreads. The WHO has also altered the coronavirus timeline on its website, now saying it got information about the virus from WHO scientists and not the Beijing authorities, as it had claimed for more than six months.

Fox News has also reached out to the Chinese Ministry of Foreign Affairs and the scientists Yan accuses of suppressing her concerns for comment. In the meantime, Yan has continued to speak the truth about the deception surrounding the virus.

A second prominent scientist who has been unafraid to call out the government deception surrounding the COVID-19 virus is virologist Dr. Judy Mikovits, who granted an interview in a viral tell-all video–Plandemic.[69]

Mikovits started her career as a lab technician at the National Cancer Institute (NCI) in 1988. She became a scientist and obtained a Ph.D. in biochemistry and molecular biology from George Washington University in 1991. By 2009, she was research director at the Whittemore Peterson Institute (WPI), a private research center in Reno, Nevada.[70]

When asked if she believed that the novel coronavirus was created in the laboratory, Mikovits said, "I wouldn't use the word 'created.' But you can't say 'naturally occurring' if it was by way of the laboratory. So it's very clear this virus was manipulated. This family of viruses was manipulated and studied in a laboratory where the animals were taken into the laboratory, and this is what was released, whether deliberate or not. That cannot be naturally occurring. Somebody didn't go to a market, get a bat; the virus didn't jump directly to humans. That's not how it works. That's accelerated viral evolution. If it was a natural occurrence, it would take up to 800 years to occur."

Mikovits suspects that the bioengineering of the virus may have occurred in one of three places: the North Carolina laboratories, the U.S. Army Medical Research Institute of Infectious Diseases at Fort Detrick, or the Wuhan laboratory.

Mikovits believes that wearing a mask activates a person's viruses. In her interview, she said, "You're getting sick from your own reactivated coronavirus expressions, and if it happens to be SARS-CoV-2, then you've got a big problem."

She also insists that closing down public places was the government's way of getting everyone sick. "Why would you close the beach? You've got sequences in the soil, in the sand. You've got healing microbes in the ocean, in the salt water. That's insanity."

Interestingly, no one has ever been able to provide satisfactory explanations as to why facemasks are necessary and why it is so important that the public wears them outdoors. According to the WHO, seasonal influenza kills up to 650,000 people every year. The infection has been around for over a hundred years, so why has everyone waited until this moment to be concerned with wearing a mask? This only proves that this mask policy is not necessarily guided by scientific evidence.[71]

Mikovitz was called a conspiracy theorist for granting this interview. Her name was tarnished all over the internet for daring to say things that other scientists were afraid to say at the time. However, today, dozens of scientists, including the WHO, have publicly stated that masks are unnecessary in preventing the spread of the virus.[72, 73, 74, 75]

A third prominent dissenting voice in the media is Dr. Rashid A. Buttar,[76] who insists that the government is hiding a lot of information about the COVID-19 pandemic and that the public needs to start digging up this information if they ever want to know the truth. Buttar is a licensed emergency medicine doctor who has been practising medicine for about 30 years.

The first coronavirus was discovered in the 1960s and it has been studied over 14,000 times since then. In all these studies, the virus was never seen to cause much of a problem and was often described as 'not a big deal' and very self-limiting. However, in 2010–2011, patents of replications of the virus started to be discovered. Dr. Buttar notes that one can only patent a virus if it's been changed, adulterated, or mutated, which means that the coronavirus was altered.[77]

According to Dr. Buttar, if you check the European Union patent database, you'll find multiple patents of the coronavirus that were already granted. One of those patents was granted in November 2019, just before the first case of COVID-19 in Wuhan. Interestingly, this 2019 patent and other patents are owned by Pirbright, an institute funded by the Bill and Melinda Gates Foundation.

It is quite interesting how Bill Gates, who is by no means a health or medical officer, has always been involved with virus research. According to Buttar, Gates "couldn't keep viruses out of Microsoft but tries to keep viruses out of the human body. As if viruses need to be kept out of the human body. Humans depend on viruses to evolve."

Bill Gates has given a lot of money to the CDC, the WHO, and many global health organizations in a bid to have a say in their research. He believes in population control and has talked about how vaccines are necessary to decrease the population.

Public health advocates around the world have accused Microsoft billionaire Bill Gates of trying to shift the focus of the World Health Organization away from hygiene, nutrition, economic development, and other projects that are proven to curb infectious diseases, and direct it towards vaccines.

Not only does Gates use his philanthropy to control global health organizations such as the WHO, UNICEF, GAVI, and PATH, he also funds a private pharmaceutical company that manufactures vaccines, and has channelled millions of dollars towards speeding up the development of a coronavirus vaccine, thereby serving his philosophy that good health only comes in a syringe.

Gates has appeared in the media recently, alluding to the idea that the COVID-19 crisis is an opportunity for him to try out his vaccine programs on American children. This has sparked outrage from health enthusiasts all around the world, some even picking up placards to embark on protest marches, as many attempt to take a stand against Big Pharma and reject mandatory vaccines.

According to the alternative medicine expert and owner of the website *Natural News*, Mike Adams, the 2019 coronavirus is a bioweapon designed in a Wuhan lab and is intended to be used to crash the world economy and achieve widespread starvation and depopulation, forcing the world into embracing vaccines.

Adams alleges that the Wuhan laboratory that created the coronavirus was receiving millions of dollars in NIH funding under the Obama administration, and that the virus is the ultimate dream of depopulation globalists like Bill Gates and Dr. Fauci.

Adams describes Gates's vaccines as "a strategic philanthropy that feed[s] his many vaccine-related businesses (including Microsoft's ambition to control a global vaccination ID enterprise) and give[s] him dictatorial control of global health policy."

Buttar accuses Gates of paying scientists to make the coronavirus worse, then being at the forefront of finding a cure and trying to force people to adopt this cure.

The United Kingdom changed its legislation on April 27, 2020 to reflect mandatory vaccines for everyone, and the entire world would follow suit in no time.

It has become apparent that the cycle is to create a problem, try to find a solution to the problem, and then force this solution on everyone. Obama had predicted that the 2009 H1N1 pandemic was going to kill 60 million Americans, but the real number of deaths ended up being 12,469 because no one took the vaccine. The public must also resist mandatory COVID-19 vaccines to prevent the government's population-control agenda.

Worse still, the truth about the COVID-19 virus is getting taken off the internet, and the government is making it hard for the public to access this information. Right now, if you say anything about 5G on Facebook or YouTube, your post will get taken down. These 5G-coronavirus videos hit millions of views before they get taken down because people feel the truth in these videos.

Buttar believes that there is a link between the 5G technology and the novel coronavirus, and that the more the government rolls out the 5G technology, the more people are going to get sick, and then they would use mandatory vaccines to make people even sicker and continue to decrease the world's population.

THE CONNECTION BETWEEN 5G
WIRELESS TECHNOLOGY AND THE
CORONAVIRUS EXPOSED

RECENTLY, THERE HAS BEEN AN overwhelming amount of evidence that shows a link between coronavirus and 5G technology. It is no coincidence that the ongoing COVID-19 pandemic that has held the world hostage all year began in Wuhan—a model city for demonstrating 5G wireless technology in China.

Since this discovery, scientists have been led to compare the crippling health effects of the 5G wireless technology to the symptoms of the coronavirus, and the results are quite grim. Scientists that study electromagnetic fields (EMF) have found that 5G deployment causes flu-like symptoms in people exposed to it.

According to Mike Adams, speaking in an interview with Alex Jones on *Infowars*, "Wuhan was the first city to install the 5G technology and look what happened there."[78]

Adams likens the ongoing pandemic to the ancient Roman Empire, which accidentally poisoned citizens by having lead-lined water pipes they thought were safe and which they embraced as a part of the city's infrastructure. Now the world has 5G towers that are blasting citizens with electromagnetic pollution. People are told that it's safe, but evidence suggests that it's not.

This doesn't mean people can't get infected with the coronavirus without being exposed to the 5G technology. It just means that it's more difficult to get infected with the virus without the electroporation/electropermeabilization effect of 5G on your body. Adams describes the duo of 5G technology and the coronavirus as a binary weapon system that combines these two factors, making it extra-dangerous and extra-real. This doesn't mean that the virus isn't real in itself; however, it is potentiated by this voltage exposure that permeates your skin.

The 5G works by sending a beam to track you. This beam follows you, goes to your phone, and penetrates your body. It's not an omni-directional signal that's being dialed everywhere; rather, it goes with you, making you more susceptible to diseases, even viruses like COVID-19.

Worse still is what 5G does to your immune system. The 5G technology puts additional pressure on the voltage gate that is designed to protect your cells and keep them in balance. This extra force throws the cells off-balance, alongside other catastrophic effects, which are sometimes irreversible. The above symptoms are similar to those that may have been felt by coronavirus patients in Wuhan.

Rather than uninstall 5G towers, the U.S. government is focused on carrying out antibody tests on people who have survived the virus and trying to find a vaccine because, to them, the profit is all that matters.

Is the Coronavirus a Bioweapon? The Answer Is YES!

Was the COVID-19 virus was manufactured to target all geopolitical and economic rivals of the United States? China and Iran are the biggest countries in this group; Italy is also a part of this group, being the first major European economy to join China's massive Belt and Road Initiative (BRI) program. Could the Italians have been targeted after they refused to back out of this deal with China?[79]

It's no news that, for over a decade now, China has been continually rising as a competitor to the United States, having embarked on many acts of financial and economic warfare against its rival. Was the virus unleashed on China in retaliation, to bring the country to its knees for the benefit of the United States?

The WHO is funded by Big Pharma and would do anything to please its biggest sponsors, hence the list of incompetent and bad advice issued at the onset of the COVID-19 outbreak.[80]

There is a lot of fear-mongering going on, targeted at getting the public to accept toxic, hastily made, experimental, extremely dangerous, and expensive vaccines that can damage the human body.[81, 82] About ten years ago, the Rockefeller Foundation published a report titled, "Scenarios for the Future of Technology and International Development."[83, 84]

One scenario carried in the report bears the captivating title, "LOCK STEP: A world of tighter top-down government control and more authoritarian leadership, with limited innovation and growing citizen pushback."

The scenario states:

"In 2012, the pandemic that the world had been anticipating for years finally hit. Unlike 2009's H1N1, this new influenza strain — originating from wild geese — was extremely virulent and deadly. Even the most pandemic-prepared nations were quickly overwhelmed when the virus streaked around the world, infecting nearly 20 percent of the global population and killing 8 million in just seven months…"

That's not all. The report continues:

"The pandemic also had a deadly effect on economies: international mobility of both people and goods screeched to a halt, debilitating industries like tourism and breaking global supply chains. Even locally, normally bustling shops and office buildings sat empty for months, devoid of both employees and customers."

Sound familiar?

Then the scenario gets even more eerie:

"During the pandemic, national leaders around the world flexed their authority and imposed airtight rules and restrictions, from the mandatory wearing of face masks to body-temperature checks at the entries to communal spaces like train stations and supermarkets. Even after the pandemic faded, this more authoritarian control and oversight of citizens and their activities stuck and even intensified. In order to protect themselves from the spread of increasingly global problems — from pandemics and transnational terrorism to environmental crises and rising poverty — leaders around the world took a firmer grip on power."

The message here is clear: "lockdown good, freedom bad."[85] Yet, studies comparing locked-down states in the United States to non-locked-down states find out the COVID-19 death toll is considerably higher in states where citizens are locked indoors for fear of the disease.[86, 87, 88, 89] In the past months, everything spelled out in this scenario has come to pass in different countries all over the world. There are limits on socialization and travel, replacement of cash transactions by electronic transactions, mandatory vaccines, constant surveillance, and a limit on personal freedom, among other restrictions.[90]

All the evidence points to the fact that fear is the perfect tool for controlling human behaviour. The public has been hyped up with so much fear and so few facts, all towards the single aim of establishing a new world order controlled by men with money.[91]

Conclusion

B ILLIONAIRE PATENT OWNERS HAVE BEGUN to push for globally mandated vaccines, as already predicted. Anyone who rejects these hastily made experimental poisons will be barred from travel, education, and work. It sounds like a horror movie, but this is today's reality.

Everyone that matters is ignoring the real issue at hand, which is that more investigation is needed to hold accountable those that are responsible for fabricating the 2019 coronavirus. Many parties involved in the pandemic have a lot to hide, which is the reason no one is calling for more investigation. From the Chinese government to the United States Centers for Disease Control and the National Institutes of Health, the World Health Organization, and the Bill and Melinda Gates Foundation, everyone would be implicated when it comes to light that the COVID-19 virus was indeed engineered at the Wuhan Institute of Virology lab. Most of the work done at the WIV was funded by U.S. taxpayers with funds channelled there by Peter Daszak and the EcoHealth Alliance.

It is interesting to note that, since the onset of the pandemic, with all the allegations faced by the WIV, they have yet to release their lab notebooks for investigation. All that would be needed to confirm the lab's guilt or innocence is a look at their lab records, staff health records, and incident reports of accidents and near-accidents.

Why has the Chinese government not released these records once and for all to clear its name? To end all questions of whether SARS-CoV-2 was engineered or passaged at the WIV lab, Zhengli Shi and Peter Daszak should prove that nothing similar to SARS-CoV-2 was being studied there by releasing those notebooks; this should ultimately absolve the lab from having knowingly made an actual pandemic pathogen.

In the absence of this kind of transparency, deep inquiries need to continue until the people responsible accept that this virus was first plucked from the wild, and then dangerous experiments were performed on it before it was unleashed on the public. The vaccine industry has discovered a 'get-even-richer-quick' scheme: this scheme involves creating a problem, intensifying fear among members of the public, and then offering a pre-planned solution for this problem.

One quick recap about 2019's pandemic: world leaders manufactured the Wuhan virus. They named it COVID-19. They predicted millions of deaths, deployed the National Guard, and built makeshift hospitals, which were expected to attend to a massive overflow of patients. They dug mass graves. They asked the public to stay at home to avoid contact with others so that the public's only news source became the internet, yet they censored what was available on the internet so that anyone who wanted to know what was really going on outside could only find the government's carefully constructed propaganda. It is time to finally open our eyes and accept the scam that has been our global health system for years. This begins by ignoring the government's narrative and embracing the truth, and that is the fact that the COVID-19 virus was indeed bioengineered in the lab for profit.

References

1. **Huang, C., Wang, Y., Li X., Ren, L., Zhao, J., Hu, Y., (2020).** Clinical features of patients infected with 2019 novel coronavirus in Wuhan, China. *The Lancet*, 395(10223), 497-506. January 24, 2020. DOI: *https://doi.org/10.1016/S0140-6736(20)30183-5*

2. **Coronavirus: Trump stands by China lab origin theory for virus.** (2020, May 1). Retrieved from *https://www.bbc.com/news/world-us-canada-52496098*

3. **Wuhan virus: China may have just accepted that the 'man-made' coronavirus escaped its biowarfare lab.** (2020, May 5). Retrieved from *https://www.ibtimes.sg/wuhan-virus-china-may-have-just-accepted-that-man-made-coronavirus-escaped-its-biowarfare-lab-39911*

4. **Don't buy China's story: The coronavirus may have leaked from a lab.** (2020, February 22). Retrieved from *https://nypost.com/2020/02/22/dont-buy-chinas-story-the-coronavirus-may-have-leaked-from-a-lab/*

5. **Was the 2020 Wuhan Coronavirus an Engineered Biological Attack on China by America for Geopolitical Advantage?** (2020, January 27). Retrieved from *https://www.unz.com/article/was-the-2020-wuhan-coronavirus-an-engineered-biological-attack-on-china-by-america-for-geopolitical-advantage/#sars-conspiracy-theory*

6. **Plandemic: Indoctornation World Premiere.** [Video File]. (2020, August 18). Retrieved from *https://freedomplatform.tv/ plandemic-indoctornation-world-premiere/*

7. **Title 35 U.S. Code § 101. Inventions patentable.** Retrieved from *https://www.govinfo.gov/content/pkg/USCODE-2011-title35/pdf/ USCODE-2011-title35-partII-chap10-sec101.pdf*

8. **Graham, T., Biological Weapons and International Law.** (2002). *Science* 295(5564), 2325. DOI: *https://science.sciencemag. org/content/295/5564/2325*

9. **Dr. Fauci Backed Controversial Wuhan Lab with U.S. Dollars for Risky Coronavirus Research.** (2020, April 28). Retrieved from *https://www.newsweek.com/dr-fauci-backed-controversial-wuhan- lab-millions-us-dollars-risky-coronavirus-research-1500741*

10. **Why Would the US Have Funded the Controversial Wuhan Lab?** (2020, May 13) Retrieved from *https://thediplomat.com/2020/05/ why-would-the-us-have-funded-the-controversial-wuhan-lab/*

11. **Andersen, K.G., Rambaut, A., Lipkin, W.I. et al:** The proximal origin of SARS-CoV-2. *Nature Medicine* 26, 450–452 (2020). DOI: *https://doi.org/10.1038/s41591-020-0820-9*

12. **Sørensen, B., Susrud, A., & Dalgleish, A.** (2020). Biovacc-19: A Candidate Vaccine for Covid-19 (SARS-CoV-2) Developed from Analysis of its General Method of Action for Infectivity. *QRB Discovery*, 1, E6. doi: 10.1017/qrd.2020.8

13. **British-Norwegian Research Study Calls Covid-19 Man-Made In China.** (2020, June 11). Retrieved from *https://enewsplanet. com/british-norwegian-research-study-calls-covid-19-man-made- in-china/*

14. **Herfst, S., Schrauwen, E. J., Linster, M., Chutinimitkul, S., de Wit, E., Munster, V. J., Sorrell, E. M., Bestebroer, T. M., Burke, D. F., Smith, D. J., Rimmelzwaan, G. F., Osterhaus, A. D., & Fouchier, R. A.** (2012). Airborne transmission of influenza A/ H5N1 virus between ferrets. *Science* (New York, N.Y.), 336(6088), 1534–1541. *https://doi.org/10.1126/science.1213362*

15. **Sheahan, T., Rockx, B., Sims, A., Raymond, P., Corti, D & Baric. R.** (2008) Mechanisms of Zoonotic Severe Acute Respiratory Syndrome Coronavirus Host Range Expansion in Human Airway Epithelium. *Journal of Virology* 82 (5), 2274-2285; DOI: 10.1128/ JVI.02041-07

16. **Butler, D.,** Engineered bat virus stirs debate over risky research (2015) *Nature* News. Retrieved from *https://www.nature.com/ news/engineered-bat-virus-stirs-debate-over-risky-research-1.18787#b1*

17. **Coutard, B., Valle, C., de Lamballerie, X., Canard, B., Seidah, N.G., & Decroly, E.** (2020) The spike glycoprotein of the new coronavirus 2019-nCoV contains a furin-like cleavage site absent in CoV of the same clade. *Antiviral Research.* 176 (104742), ISSN 0166-3542. *https://doi.org/10.1016/j.antiviral.2020.104742*

18. **How Could a Virus be Genetically Engineered?** (2020) Retrieved from *https://www.news-medical.net/health/How-Could-a-Virus-be-Genetically-Engineered.aspx*

19. **Ex-head of MI6 Sir Richard Dearlove says coronavirus 'is man-made' and was 'released by accident'–after seeing 'important' scientific report.** (2020, June 4) Retrieved from *https://www. dailymail.co.uk/news/article-8386235/Coronavirus-man-says-ex-head-MI6-Sir-Richard-Dearlove.html*

20. **Fauci dismisses Trump's coronavirus Wuhan lab claims.** (2020, May 5) Retrieved from *https://www.aljazeera.com/ news/2020/5/5/fauci-dismisses-trumps-coronavirus-wuhan-lab-claims*

21. **Hu, B., Zeng, L.-P., Yang, X.-L., Ge, X.-Y., Zhang, W., Li, B., et al.** (2017) Discovery of a rich gene pool of bat SARS-related coronaviruses provides new insights into the origin of SARS coronavirus. *PLOS Pathogens* 13(11): e1006698. *https://doi. org/10.1371/journal.ppat.1006698*

22. **Zhan, S.H., Deverman, B.E., & Chan, Y.A.** (2020) SARS-CoV-2 is well adapted for humans. What does this mean for

re-emergence? *bioRxiv* 2020.05.01.073262; doi: *https://doi.org/10.1101/2020.05.01.073262*

23. **Zhou, P., Yang, X., Wang, X. et al.** (2020). A pneumonia outbreak associated with a new coronavirus of probable bat origin. *Nature* 579, 270–273 *https://doi.org/10.1038/s41586-020-2012-7*

24. **Ge, X., Li, J., Yang, X. et al.** (2013). Isolation and characterization of a bat SARS-like coronavirus that uses the ACE2 receptor. *Nature* 503, 535–538. DOI: *https://doi.org/10.1038/nature12711*

25. **Wan, Y., Shang, J., Graham R., Baric, R. S., & Li, F.,** (2020). Receptor Recognition by the Novel Coronavirus from Wuhan: an Analysis Based on Decade-Long Structural Studies of SARS Coronavirus. *Journal of Virology*, 94 (7) e00127-20; DOI: 10.1128/JVI.00127-20

26. **History of 1918 Flu Pandemic: Centers for Disease Control and Prevention.** Retrieved from *https://www.cdc.gov/flu/pandemic-resources/1918-commemoration/1918-pandemic-history.htm*

27. **Nakajima, K., Desselberger, U., & Palese, P.** (1978). Recent human influenza A (H1N1) viruses are closely related genetically to strains isolated in 1950. *Nature* 274, 334–339. *https://doi.org/10.1038/274334a0*

28. **Duggal, A., Pinto, R., Rubenfeld, G., & Fowler, R. A.** (2016). Global variability in reported mortality for critical illness during the 2009-10 influenza A (H1N1) pandemic: a systematic review and meta-regression to guide reporting of outcomes during disease outbreaks. *PLOS ONE*, 11(5), e0155044.

29. **Simonsen, L., Spreeuwenberg, P., Lustig, R., Taylor, R. J., Fleming, D. M., Kroneman, M., & Paget, W. J.** (2013). Global mortality estimates for the 2009 Influenza Pandemic from the GLaMOR project: a modeling study. *PLOS Medicine*, 10(11), e1001558.

30. **Wertheim, J. O.** (2010). The re-emergence of H1N1 influenza virus in 1977: a cautionary tale for estimating divergence times using biologically unrealistic sampling dates. *PLOS ONE*, 5(6), e11184.

31. **The Case is Building that Covid-19 had a Lab Origin.** (2020, June 19). Retrieved from *https://www.independentsciencenews. org/health/the-case-is-building-that-covid-19-had-a-lab-origin/*

32. **Furmanski, M.** (2014). Laboratory Escapes and "Self-fulfilling prophecy" Epidemics. *Report: Center for Arms Control and Nonproliferation.* PDF available online.

33. **Lipsitch M.** (2018). "Why Do Exceptionally Dangerous Gain-of-Function Experiments in Influenza?". In Yamauchi, Y. (eds) *Influenza Virus.* Methods in Molecular Biology (Clifton, N.J.), 1836, 589–608. *https://doi.org/10.1007/978-1-4939-8678-1_29*

34. **Klotz, L. C., & Sylvester, E. J.** (2014). The consequences of a lab escape of a potential pandemic pathogen. *Frontiers in Public Health*, 2, 116. *https://doi.org/10.3389/fpubh.2014.00116*

35. **1994 Surat Plague – A Forgotten Case Of Bioterrorism.** (2020, July 2). Available at *https://greatgameindia.com/1994-surat-plague-bioterrorism/*

36. **Human error in high-biocontainment labs: a likely pandemic threat.** (2019, February 25). Retrieved from *https://thebulletin. org/2019/02/human-error-in-high-biocontainment-labs-a-likely-pandemic-threat/*

37. **Weiss, S., Yitzhaki, S., & Shapira, S. C.** (2015). Lessons to be Learned from Recent Biosafety Incidents in the United States. *The Israel Medical Association Journal: IMAJ*, 17(5), 269-273. Available at *https://pubmed.ncbi.nlm.nih.gov/26137650/*

38. **Hu, B., Zeng, L.-P., Yang, X.-L., Ge, X.-Y., Zhang, W., Li, B., et al.** (2017). Discovery of a rich gene pool of bat SARS-related coronaviruses provides new insights into the origin of SARS coronavirus. *PLOS Pathogens*, 13(11), e1006698. *https://doi. org/10.1371/journal.ppat.1006698*

39. **Zhou, P., Yang, X. L., Wang, X. G., Hu, B., Zhang, L., Zhang, W., & Chen, H. D.** (2020). A pneumonia outbreak associated with a new coronavirus of probable bat origin. *Nature*, 579(7798), 270-273. *https://doi.org/10.1038/s41586-020-2012-7*

40. **Scientific evidence and logic behind the claim that the Wuhan coronavirus is man-made.** (2020 March 15). Available at *https://nerdhaspower.weebly.com/blog/scientific-evidence-and-logic-behind-the-claim-that-the-wuhan-coronavirus-is-man-made*

41. **Wrapp D., Wang, K. S., Corbett, S. K., Goldsmith, A. J., Hsieh, C., Abiona, O., Graham, S., Mclellan J.S** (2020) Cryo-EM structure of the 2019-nCoV spike in the prefusion conformation. *Science* 367 (6483) 1260-1263 *DOI: 10.1126/science.abb2507*

42. **Zhang, T., Wu, Q., Zhang, Z.** (2020). Probable Pangolin Origin of 2019-nCoV Associated with Outbreak of COVID-19. Available at SSRN: *https://ssrn.com/abstract=3542586* or *http://dx.doi.org/10.2139/ssrn.3542586*

43. **Zeng, L., Gao, Y., Ge, X., Zhang, Q., Peng Cheng, Yang, X., Tan, B., Chen, J., Chmura, A., Daszak, P. & Shi, Z.** (2016). Bat Severe Acute Respiratory Syndrome-Like Coronavirus WIV1 Encodes an Extra Accessory Protein, ORFX, Involved in Modulation of the Host Immune Response. *Journal of Virology*, 90 (14) 6573-6582; DOI: *10.1128/JVI.03079-15*

44. **Li, W., Shi, Z., Yu, M., Ren, W., Smith, C., Epstein, J.H., Wang, H., Crameri, G., Hu, Z., Zhang, H., Zhang, J., McEachern, J., Field, H., Daszak, P., Eaton, B.T., Zhang, S., & Wang, L.-F.** (2005). Bats are natural reservoirs of SARS-like coronaviruses. *Science* 310 (5748): 676-9. doi: *10.1126/science.1118391*

45. **Ge, X.-Y., Wang, N., Zhang, W., Hu, B., Li, B., Zhang, Y.-Z., Zhou, J.-H., Luo, C.-M., Yang, X.-L., Wu, L.-J., Wang, B., Zhang, Y., Li, Z.-X., & Shi, Z.-L.** (2013). Coexistence of multiple coronaviruses in several bat colonies in an abandoned mineshaft. *Virologica Sinica* 1(1): 31-40. doi: *10.1007/s12250-016-3713-9*

46. **Hu, B., Ge, X., Wang, L. et al.** (2015). Bat origin of human coronaviruses. *Journal of Virology* 12, 221. *https://doi.org/10.1186/s12985-015-0422-1*

47. **Menachery, V. D., Yount, B. L., Debbink, K., Agnihothram, S., Gralinski, L. E., Plante, J. A., ... & Randell, S. H.** (2015). A

SARS-like cluster of circulating bat coronaviruses shows potential for human emergence. *Nature Medicine*, 21(12), 1508-1513.

48. **Wrapp, D., Wang, N., Corbett, K. S., Goldsmith, J. A., Hsieh, C. L., Abiona, O., ... & McLellan, J. S.** (2020). Cryo-EM structure of the 2019-nCoV spike in the prefusion conformation. *Science*, 367(6483), 1260-1263.

49. **Wan, Y., Shang, J., Graham, R., Baric, R. S., & Li, F.** (2020). Receptor recognition by the novel coronavirus from Wuhan: an analysis based on decade-long structural studies of SARS coronavirus. *Journal of Virology*, 94 (7), e00127-20. DOI: 10.1128/JVI.00127-20

50. **Letko, M., Marzi, A. & Munster.** (2020). Functional assessment of cell entry and receptor usage for SARS-CoV-2 and other lineage B betacoronaviruses. *Nature Microbiology* 5, 562–569. *https://doi.org/10.1038/s41564-020-0688-y*

51. **Piplani, S., Singh, P. K, Winkler, D. A., Petrovsky, N.** (2020) In silico comparison of spike protein-ACE2 binding affinities across species; significance for the possible origin of the SARS-CoV-2 virus. *arXiv.org > q-bio > arXiv:2005.06199*

52. **Did the SARS-CoV-2 virus arise from a bat coronavirus research program in a Chinese laboratory? Very possibly.** (2020, June 4) Available at *https://thebulletin.org/2020/06/did-the-sars-cov-2-virus-arise-from-a-bat-coronavirus-research-program-in-a-chinese-laboratory-very-possibly/*

53. **Irrefutable: The Coronavirus Was Engineered by Scientists in a Lab Using Well Documented Genetic Engineering Vectors That Leave Behind a "Fingerprint".** (2020, February 3). Available at *http://theunhivedmind.com/news/2020/02/04/irrefutable-the-coronavirus-was-engineered-by-scientists-in-a-lab-using-well-documented-genetic-engineering-vectors-that-leave-behind-a-fingerprint/*

54. **Lu, R., Zhao, X., Li, J., Niu, P., Yang, B., Wu, H.,** (2020) Genomic characterisation and epidemiology of 2019 novel coronavirus: implications for virus origins and receptor binding. *The Lancet*,

395 (10224), pp.565-574. DOI: *https://www.thelancet.com/article/S0140-6736%2820%2930251-8/fulltext*

55. **EXPERT REACTION: Did COVID-19 come from a lab in Wuhan?** (2020, April 17). Available at *https://www.scimex.org/newsfeed/expert-reaction-did-covid-19-come-from-a-lab-in-wuhan*

56. **Coronavirus: Man-Made, Bill Gates and Madonna.** (2019, November 4). Available from *https://www.whatsorb.com/community/coronavirus-bill-gates-65-million-death-in-a-simulation*

57. **Australian researchers see virus design manipulation.** (2020, May 21). Available at: *https://www.palmerfoundation.com.au/australian-researchers-see-virus-design-manipulation/*

58. **Pradhan, P., Pandey, A.K., Mishra, A., Gupta, P., Tripathi, P.K., Menon, M.B., Gomes, J., Vivekanandan, P., & Kundu, B.** (2020). Uncanny similarity of unique inserts in the 2019-nCoV spike protein to HIV-1 gp120 and Gag. doi: 10.1101/2020.01.30.927871

59. **Sirotkin, K., & Sirotkin, J.** (2020). Might SARS-CoV-2 Have Arisen via Serial Passage through an Animal Host or Cell Culture? A potential explanation for much of the novel coronavirus' distinctive genome. Available at *https://onlinelibrary.wiley.com/doi/epdf/10.1002/bies.202000091*

60. **How does coronavirus kill? Clinicians trace a ferocious rampage through the body, from brain to toes.** (2020, April 17). Available at *https://www.sciencemag.org/news/2020/04/how-does-coronavirus-kill-clinicians-trace-ferocious-rampage-through-body-brain-toes*

61. **Yes, coronavirus is a BIOWEAPON with gene sequencing that's only possible if it was genetically modified in a lab.** (2020, February 11). Available at: *https://thecommonsenseshow.com/conspiracy-health-martial-law/yes-coronavirus-bioweapon-gene-sequencing-thats-only-possible-if-it-was-genetically-modified-lab*

62. **How China's 'Bat Woman' Hunted Down Viruses from SARS**

to the New Coronavirus. (2020, June 1). Available at: *https://www.scientificamerican.com/article/how-chinas-bat-woman-hunted-down-viruses-from-sars-to-the-new-coronavirus1/*

63. Bill Gates Calls for a "Digital Certificate" to Identify Who Received COVID-19 Vaccine. (2020, April 1). Available at: *https://vigilantcitizen.com/latestnews/bill-gates-calls-for-a-digital-certificate-to-identify-who-is-vaccinated/*

64. Passport to the Brave New World: the vaccine. (2020, April 14). Available at: *https://blog.nomorefakenews.com/2020/04/14/passport-to-the-brave-new-world-the-vaccine/*

65. Coronavirus Update with Anthony S. Fauci, MD. [Video File] (2020 September, 25). Available at: *https://www.youtube.com/watch?v=R84Rvcc9mu0*

66. Protection Without a Vaccine. (2015, March 9). Available at: *https://www.nytimes.com/2015/03/10/health/protection-without-a-vaccine.html*

67. David Baltimore: Broad Institute. Available at *https://www.broadinstitute.org/what-broad/history-leadership/board-scientific-counselors/bios/david-baltimore-phd*

68. EXCLUSIVE: Chinese virologist accuses Beijing of coronavirus cover-up, flees Hong Kong: 'I know how they treat whistleblowers.' (2020, July 10). Available at *https://www.foxnews.com/world/chinese-virologist-coronavirus-cover-up-flee-hong-kong-whistleblower*

69. Plandemic: Indoctornation. (2020). Available at *https://plandemicseries.com/*

70. Fact-checking Judy Mikovits, the controversial virologist attacking Anthony Fauci in a viral conspiracy video. (2020, May 8). Available at *https://www.sciencemag.org/news/2020/05/fact-checking-judy-mikovits-controversial-virologist-attacking-anthony-fauci-viral*

71. World Health Organization: Influenza Are We Ready?

Available at *https://www.who.int/news-room/spotlight/influenza-are-we-ready*

72. **Science Says Healthy People Should NOT Wear Masks.** (2020, July 26). Available at *https://principia-scientific.com/science-says-healthy-people-should-not-wear-masks/*

73. **Commentary: In Mask Debate, Social Distancing Remains Priority.** (2020, April 2). Available at *https://publichealth.uic.edu/news-stories/commentary-masks-for-all-for-covid-19-not-based-on-sound-data/*

74. **WHO stands by recommendation to not wear masks if you are not sick or not caring for someone who is sick.** (2020, March 21). Available at *https://edition.cnn.com/2020/03/30/world/coronavirus-who-masks-recommendation-trnd/index.html*

75. **The surgeon general wants Americans to stop buying face masks.** (2020, March 2). Available at *https://www.cnn.com/2020/02/29/health/face-masks-coronavirus-surgeon-general-trnd/index.html*

76. **Doximity: Dr. Rashid Ali Buttar.** Available at *https://www.doximity.com/pub/rashid-buttar-do*

77. **Dr. Rashid Buttar: What We Need to Know.** [Video File] (2020, May 1). Available at: *https://www.youtube.com/watch?v=gIy4QgsvryQ*

78. **Infowars: Alex Jones.** Available at *https://www.liveleak.com/view?t=CIM4m_1586160635*

79. **OPERATION LOCK-STEP – The Sinister Agenda behind Covid-19.** (2020, March 10). Available at *https://behind-the-news.com/operation-lock-step-the-sinister-agenda-behind-covid-19/*

80. **World Health Organization Faces Calls for Leader to Resign over Coronavirus Failure.** (2020, March 26). Available at: *https://www.breitbart.com/national-security/2020/03/26/world-health-organization-faces-calls-for-leader-to-resign-over-coronavirus-failure/*

81. **Dozens of COVID-19 vaccines are in development. Here are the ones to follow.** (2020, October 2). Available at: *https://*

www.nationalgeographic.com/science/health-and-human-body/
human-diseases/coronavirus-vaccine-tracker-how-they-work-
latest-developments-cvd/

82. **Visualizing the Secret History Of Coronavirus Bioweapon.**
(2020, March 16). Available at: *https://greatgameindia.com/*
secret-history-of-coronavirus-bioweapon/

83. **Scenarios for the Future of Technology and International**
Development. (2010). Available at *https://www.academia.*
*edu/42295029/Rockefeller_Vakf%C4%B1n%C4%B1n_*
*May%C4%B1s_2010_Raporu_Scenarios_for_the_Future_of_*
*Technology_and_International_Development_*

84. **The Rockefeller Foundation: Scenarios for the Future of**
Technology and International Development. (2010). Available
at *https://www.nommeraadio.ee/meedia/pdf/RRS/Rockefeller%20*
Foundation.pdf

85. **Post Lockdown – The Rockefeller Game Plan Part 1.** (2020, May
10). Available at: *https://behind-the-news.com/post-lockdown-the-*
rockefeller-game-plan-part-1-of-a-2-part-series/

86. **COVID19: A Controlled Study.** (2020, March 24). Available
at: *https://colleenhuber.com/covid19-a-controlled-study/?fbclid=*
*IwAR3XrTDUVz_qVjHbBk3A2DFKp4mF1XFnQuA_*
FP9hWbQaFJ0OL1G3IqOEjas

87. **Rancourt, D.** (2020). All-cause mortality during COVID-19: No
plague and a likely signature of mass homicide by government
response. doi: 10.13140/RG.2.2.24350.77125

88. **States That Reopened Do Not Have More COVID-19 Infections**
Than Ones That Stayed Closed. (2020, May 14). Available at:
https://nationalfile.com/states-that-reopened-do-not-have-more-
covid-19-infections-than-ones-that-stayed-closed/

89. **Where Does Brian Kemp Go For an Apology?** (2020, May 14).
https://ewerickson.substack.com/p/where-does-brian-kemp-go-for-
an-apology?fbclid=IwAR04O9KM4DJ8p98YgIbS9zl-SZtBXheIpSE-
6eb8q2sQFmnzoqcHFrPp9N8

90. **Post Lockdown – The Rockefeller Game Plan Part 2 [of a 2 Part Series]**. (2020, June 10). *https://behind-the-news.com/post-lockdown-the-rockefeller-game-plan-part-2-of-a-2-part-series/*

91. **DNA, Vaccines, and Transhumanism.** (2020, October 4). *https://vaxxter.com/dna_vaccines_transhumanism/*